Saturated Facts

Dr Idrees Mughal (Dr Idz) is an NHS doctor with a master's degree in nutritional research and board certification in lifestyle medicine. As a passionate advocate of preventative healthcare, he shares informative videos on his hugely popular TikTok, Instagram and Facebook accounts to help combat the most damaging and unscientific health advice available online. Dr Mughal lives in the West Midlands with his family.

Saturated Facts

A Myth-busting Guide to Diet and Nutrition in a World of Misinformation

DR IDREES MUGHAL

PENGUIN LIFE

AN IMPRINT OF

PENGUIN BOOKS

PENGUIN LIFE

UK | USA | Canada | Ireland | Australia
India | New Zealand | South Africa

Penguin Life is part of the Penguin Random House group of companies
whose addresses can be found at global.penguinrandomhouse.com.

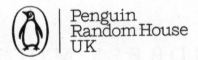

First published 2024

004

The information in this book has been compiled as general guidance on the specific subjects addressed. It is not a substitute and not to be relied on for medical, healthcare or pharmaceutical professional advice. Please consult your GP before changing, stopping or starting any medical treatment. So far as the author is aware the information given is correct and up to date as at 25 October 2023. Practice, laws and regulations all change and the reader should obtain up-to-date professional advice on any such issues. The author and publishers disclaim, as far as the law allows, any liability arising directly or indirectly from the use or misuse of the information contained in this book.

Names and identifying details have been changed. Any resemblance to actual persons is entirely coincidental.

Set in 12/14.75pt Dante MT Std
Typeset by Jouve (UK), Milton Keynes
Printed and bound in Great Britain by Clays Ltd, Elcograf S.p.A.

The authorized representative in the EEA is Penguin Random House Ireland,
Morrison Chambers, 32 Nassau Street, Dublin D02 YH68

A CIP catalogue record for this book is available from the British Library

ISBN: 978-0-241-58822-2

www.greenpenguin.co.uk

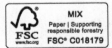

To my cherished family and friends, whose unwavering support
has been my anchor – most especially to my mother,
who has been my guiding light.

Contents

Introduction

Today's health landscape

Does *when* we eat matter for health? Is weight loss as simple as calories in versus calories out? Do carbs make you fat? Is gluten inflammatory? Is dairy dangerous? Does all disease start in the gut?

We are exposed to a growing amount of contradictory health information on the internet and social media every day. Absolutely anyone can share their opinions with millions of people at the simple touch of a button – no medical qualifications required. Every minute, new fads, hacks and trends are added to the already overwhelming quantity of advice available. The reality is that more than 60 per cent of people in the UK look to the internet for health advice,[1] yet our lives have become saturated with 'facts' about our health that are doing more harm than good. We know that false or novel-sounding information often receives more traction online – and so every day, more misinformation and fearmongering find their way onto the internet. It has been calculated that 70 per cent of research studies assessing the validity of health information online conclude that it lacks accuracy, comprehensiveness and quality.[2] Finding practical, evidence-based health advice is becoming more difficult all the time.

This isn't your typical health or nutrition book. It's not filled to the brim with low-calorie recipes, nor is it a breakdown of what a carbohydrate or a protein is. And it most definitely is *not* a book pushing the narrative that going keto is the way to live forever. I mean, what's the point of living forever if I can't eat rice again? Instead, *Saturated Facts* is a book designed for the individual who wants a comprehensive one-stop shop for how diet truly impacts our health, and a myth-busting corrective to the poor information you'll find on social media.

Preventative medicine

It wasn't until I was studying for my master's in nutritional research that I noticed the level of disconnect between nutrition education and our health. During this time, I spent twelve months working with the TwinsUK cohort, a study of more than 15,000 twins across the country. I was able to analyse millions of data points and further educate myself on various fascinating subjects, like whether diet impacts the risk of depression and other mental health disorders.

But throughout medical school, I kept thinking to myself: *Isn't it amazing how healthcare professionals only seem to care or act once someone is ill? Why don't we help people to stop them from getting these illnesses in the first place?* This led me towards preventative medicine and eventually becoming board-certified in lifestyle medicine, where we help educate people to make better lifestyle decisions and keep them from having to interact with the healthcare system in the first place.

Preventative medicine is a recognized and established medical specialty in the US, but it is still fairly small in the UK. I want to change that. I see this book as the beginning of a preventative revolution, one where we start taking our health into our own hands. We can learn so much about how to prevent and manage disease by thinking about what we put into our mouths. But first, I'll tell you a little bit about how I came to communicate this message through social media.

Social media doctor

Being online was always a daunting concept for me. I was scared that social media was no place for medical professionals, and paranoid about being judged or aggressively confronted by the latest 'Keto Karen'. These thoughts kept me away until the January 2021 COVID-19 lockdown in the UK, when I experienced a 'light bulb' moment.

I was spending ten-hour days in a hospital ward dedicated to COVID-19 patients, coming back exhausted each night to my small flat in the quaint city of Norwich. Like so many people during the pandemic I spent a lot of time alone, scrolling through TikTok in the evening, watching pranksters mess with drive-through employees or seeing people learn the latest dance trend. Then, one day, I stumbled across a video with 10 million views.

It was titled 'lose 10lbs in 2 WEEKS!' My bullsh** senses were already tingling. The video featured a woman dressed in the latest fitness gear, showing viewers how to craft a juice blend of cucumber, pineapple and lemon water that would supposedly aid with weight loss. Perhaps the most concerning part was the thousands of comments from viewers saying they were going to start the regimen that same day! I commented, pleading with people not to engage with this juice diet, only for my attempts to be engulfed by the virality of the video.

I remember feeling a volatile mix of amusement and fear as I watched medical falsehood after falsehood be perpetuated online. I'd feel almost traumatized when I saw what was trending in the health conversation (ten-day water fasts, ketone supplements, coffee enemas). Eventually, I felt compelled and morally obligated to do something in the name of health and science. I pondered for hours on how I could benefit social media from both a healthcare and personal wellness perspective. I wanted to reach more than just the patients I saw each day at the hospital. And perhaps through my efforts, I could even help to decrease the number of people in hospitals altogether.

I was sure that I *could* make a difference, if only I had a large enough platform to fight back against the pseudoscience devil laughing hysterically at me, daring me to make my move. So, I dipped my toes in the murky waters of social media and started recording humorous videos, just to get a flavour of how the public would respond. I covered a range of themes, like the struggles of working out during lockdown and making the life-changing decision of whether to 'bulk' or 'cut'. My early posts weren't always calculated or precise, but those initial few weeks allowed me to become comfortable putting myself out there in the public eye. My anxiety slowly diminished as I strategically planned my first educational video titled 'Stop telling people a calorie is a calorie' and then posted it.

Just a few months later, I was getting tagged in hundreds of videos each and every day, with requests for feedback on all kinds of health- and nutrition-related topics. That's when I realized I'd found my calling. My audience wanted me to debunk these fear-mongering health 'gurus', breaking down the research to sift fact from fiction, and I was only too happy to oblige.

How to use this book

Saturated Facts has the same goal as my social media posts – to myth-bust, inform and educate. It isn't about me. It's about empowering *you* to make informed decisions about your own health, underpinned by real nutritional research.

Let me ask you something. If I took you aside and said: 'If you take this tablet every day, your risk of dying prematurely will decrease by 20 per cent', would you be interested? But wait – it gets even better. If you take two of the tablets, your risk of dying prematurely will decrease by a further 20 per cent. Sounds too good to be true, right? And yet it actually doesn't stop there, because you could take four of these tablets daily, and each additional one would reduce your risk of dying early further still. You'd probably bite my arm off.

Well, guess what? Those 'tablets' really exist, and they each represent 1,000 *steps of walking*. Compared to no steps, a systematic review of seventeen studies found that walking just 1,000 steps a day decreases the risk of dying by 6–36 per cent over the ten-year follow-up period.[3]

The same dose-dependent relationship can be said of specific foods and patterns of eating. In fact, what we put into our mouths is arguably even *more* important for health and longevity. And so, through this book, I am going to prescribe you something life-saving. The only difference here is that the medicine doesn't come from a pharmacy – you can buy it yourself in the supermarket. The benefit of this prescription won't be seen within hours or days like in hospital, and nor does it replace life-saving pharmaceuticals. But this 'pill' will help to prevent you needing those pharmaceuticals in the first place, and will enable a better recovery if you were ever to need them.

Many so-called professionals misrepresent information to substantiate whatever narrative they may profit from financially. This is often seen with people who promote intermittent fasting or the ketogenic diet, for example. I, on the other hand, absolutely do not care which dietary habit you choose to follow. My passion is ensuring that your choice is an informed one.

That is my sole purpose with this book. No nonsense. No BS. No 'detox cleansing powders'. I will use my expertise in human physiology, health and research analysis to debunk a lot of the common wellness claims we all see circulating online, and give you the real low-down on nutrition, weight loss and health. This is a manual for everything you need to know about the role that nutrition plays in our health. And, boy, is it a BIG role! I will critically review the latest scientific evidence and explain what practical steps we can take to optimize our health.

I hope that this book will enable you to navigate your way through this world of saturated facts. So, without further ado, let's tackle some of the most prevalent diet myths we see today.

PART ONE

Common Diet Myths

Truth and Lies

From the notion that carbs make you fat, to the widely held belief that intermittent fasting is the cure to the obesity crisis, our understanding of nutrition is often clouded by a torrent of half-truths and misunderstood science. This chapter will illuminate the twisted corridors of dietary folklore, unmasking the most pervasive myths that have woven their way into the fabric of our dietary habits. Together, we'll debunk common diet myths and reveal the powerful, health-promoting truths that lie beneath them. Strap in and prepare to have your food beliefs flipped, stirred and healthily sautéed as we venture forth into the realm of dietary reality.

Diet myth no. 1: Carbs are best avoided

Far back in the hallowed halls of history, there emerged a dietary approach that would come to defy convention, spark debates and kindle a nutritional revolution: the ketogenic diet. It all began when, over 2,000 years ago, the ancient Greeks discovered that fasting could reduce the frequency and intensity of certain kinds of seizures. It was a first, vague hint of the therapeutic potential of a metabolism not fuelled by carbohydrates, though it would take many centuries before this understanding was refined into a practical treatment.

Fast-forward to 1921, when Dr Rollin Woodyatt, an endocrinologist, discovered that fasting produced not only glucose, but also two other compounds, namely acetone and beta-hydroxy-butyric acid. He realized that these are what we now know as ketone bodies – the namesake of the ketogenic diet. A couple of years later, in 1923, a man named Dr Russell Wilder proposed the ketogenic diet as a less drastic alternative to fasting, to treat pharmacoresistant epilepsy in children. Much to his delight, it worked.[1]

More recently though, the diet has been advertised as a weight-loss wonder relevant to anyone looking to lose a few pounds, as well as a treatment for type 2 diabetes. The ketogenic diet is typically characterized by high fat, adequate protein and very low carbohydrate intake (<20g). Low-carb, high-protein diets often gain attention in the fitness world – the paleo and Atkins diets fit into a similar category – but a true keto diet centres on fat, which accounts for up to 90 per cent of total energy. The keto diet aims to force your body into using a different kind of fuel. Instead of using glucose drawn from carbohydrates, it relies on the ketone bodies that are produced by the liver when stored fat is broken down, hence the name 'keto'.

When carbohydrates are broken down into glucose molecules, the main role of insulin is to transport glucose out of the blood into neighbouring cells. Here it can act as an immediate energy source for cells, or it can be stored as glycogen or fat when glucose is abundant. Simultaneously, insulin signals to the body to stop breaking down fat so it can focus on the energy coming in.

Those who promote the keto diet have grasped hold of this science but misunderstand it at the cellular level. Their theory goes: carbohydrates cause insulin levels to rise, insulin promotes fat storage and prevents fat breakdown independent of calorie intake, thus people gain weight and become hungrier. Many low-carb advocates refer to this as the Carbohydrate-Insulin Model of Obesity (CIM). While at some level it would appear to make sense that suppressing the hormone largely responsible for fat storage would be the key to weight-loss success, unfortunately the strongest of metabolic ward studies (where participants are admitted to a heavily controlled ward) prove otherwise.[2] When protein and calories are matched in both diet groups, although you'll see rapid weight loss from the loss of water from going keto (as 1g of carbs carries with it 3–4g of water), low-carb diets don't offer superior fat-loss effects over higher-carb diets.

Understanding weight gain

When it comes to understanding weight gain, scientists have two main theories. One is called the Energy Balance Model (EBM), and the other is the Carbohydrate-Insulin Model (CIM). Both theories propose that weight change happens based on the law of thermodynamics. Simply put, if you consume more energy (calories) than you burn, you gain weight.

According to the EBM, which most scientists agree on, the main reason people gain weight is that they eat too many calories, no matter what kind of food these calories come from. Factors that influence someone's calorie intake include: food processing level, taste, water content of food, fibre and so on. On the other hand, the CIM theory suggests that it's not just about how many calories you eat, but what *type* of calories. Specifically, it claims that eating carbohydrates makes your body release the hormone insulin. Insulin helps your body store fat and makes you want to eat more, which leads to weight gain.

However, people who promote low-carb or keto diets may have fundamentally misunderstood the CIM. I've heard it said that eating carbohydrates stops your body from burning fat, no matter how few calories you eat. This is not accurate. The CIM doesn't dispute the law of thermodynamics or the idea that consuming too many calories leads to weight gain.[3] Instead, it suggests a slightly different sequence of events. According to the CIM, eating carbohydrates leads to hormonal and cellular changes that make you eat more, and therefore you gain weight. It's like when a child goes through a growth spurt. The body's changes prompt the child to eat more as they grow, not before.

In a nutshell, both theories agree that consuming more energy than you burn leads to weight gain. The EBM suggests any excess calories can cause weight gain, while the CIM suggests that carbs might lead to hormonal changes that make you eat more, causing weight gain. However, in the following section we'll explain why you *don't* need to fear carbs and why the ketogenic diet is overall *not* a sensible approach for most.

Why carbs aren't the enemy

If carbs were really the problem, then wouldn't vegetarians and vegans who typically rely much more on carbohydrate-rich foods for nourishment suffer from a higher incidence of obesity, heart disease and diabetes? In fact, almost every large-scale population study that assesses dietary patterns points to a consensus that high-carb plant-based eaters have lower body weights, BMIs and risks of chronic disease. Just take the European Prospective Investigation into Cancer and Nutrition Oxford (EPIC-Oxford) study that assessed tens of thousands of people as one example. It found that, on average, vegans have far lower BMIs compared to meat eaters.[4]

A European meta-analysis of over 800,000 people found that vegans and vegetarians had a 15–21 per cent reduced risk of cardiovascular disease.[5] The same can be seen among the five longest-living populations in the world – referred to as the 'Blue Zones'. Inhabitants of these areas (which include Okinawa in Japan, Sardinia in Italy, and the Greek island of Ikaria) reach the age of 100 at rates ten times higher than people in, for example, the US as a whole,[6] and one thing they've got in common is that they've thrived on plant-based, carb-centric diets (which are rich in whole grains, greens, potatoes and beans) for centuries.

The issue with the carbophobic mindset is that it doesn't distinguish between refined, heavily processed carbohydrates like sweets, white breads and chocolate eclairs and nutritious and beneficial sources such as fruit,[7] whole grains[8] and legumes[9] (which are all independently linked to a neutral or reduction effect in weight). Obviously not all carbohydrates are equal, and there are many nutritious and filling options to choose from.

Following a ketogenic diet can have some benefits for certain people. It is clearly an effective strategy for losing weight in the short term, and also for managing type 2 diabetes.[10] Within the first 6–12 months of starting the ketogenic diet, we tend to see decreases in body weight and blood pressure, and beneficial effects on certain liver markers such as triglycerides and HDL (the 'good' cholesterol).[11] However, the aforementioned effects are generally not seen after twelve months of therapy, and there are several pretty drastic downsides to this way of eating.

The risks of a keto diet

Firstly, if you're not eating a wide variety of vegetables, fruits and grains, you'll be at a much greater risk of nutrient deficiencies such as vitamins B and C, selenium and magnesium, which could lead to fatigue, muscle weakness, mood changes and ulcers.[12] Secondly, a diet is only useful if you can actually stick to it. Many of us will have direct experience of or know someone who has tried the keto diet, lost a significant amount of weight but subsequently put it back on, only to repeat the dieting cycle over and over again. The undeniable fact is that the desire for carb-rich foods eventually wins out for most. We could save ourselves a lot of time, money and stress by learning how to incorporate more nutritious sources of carbohydrates into our diet – ones that would aid a weight-loss or healthful journey – instead of vilifying them. Viewing whole food groups as either 'good' or 'bad' falls under the term 'dichotomous beliefs' and has its own detrimental effects, which we'll cover in the chapter on 'Weight Loss: Achieving Sustainability'.

Arguably the most serious consequence of the ketogenic diet, though, is its effect on the liver. With so much fat to metabolize, the diet has the potential to negatively impact liver functionality and make any existing liver conditions worse. While restricting an entire macronutrient *could* aid in short-term weight loss, thus benefitting overweight individuals with weight-loss-associated health improvements, going keto for any prolonged period of time can have dire consequences. In one tightly controlled ketogenic feeding trial, where all meals were provided to normal-weighted women, the subjects had their urine, blood and ketone body levels tested to assess dietary adherence.[13] Following four weeks of the ketogenic diet, deleterious effects were observed on blood lipid profiles, in particular worsening LDL ('bad' cholesterol that is highly atherogenic, i.e. promoting the formation of fatty deposits in the arteries) and Apolipoprotein-B (the protein that carries LDL around the body and deposits it in arterial walls) – markers that are strongly linked to increased cardiovascular disease.*[14]

Until recently, most medical findings on low-carb keto-style diets have only been from short-term controlled trials, which has allowed keto advocates to fend off concerns. However, we are now starting to see the potential harmful effects of this diet play out in long-term observational research. In one study which spanned a decade, data from almost 500,000 people in Japan, Greece, Sweden and the US, with differing dietary patterns, was pooled together. Researchers found that people following diets that were lower in carbohydrates had a 22 per cent increased risk of earlier death, a 35 per cent increased risk of cardiovascular-related death and an 8 per cent increased risk of death from

---

* Keeping LDL low is so important that the European Atherosclerosis Society released a Consensus Panel statement in 2017, where they analysed over 200 cohort studies, Mendelian randomization and RCT studies of over 2 million people and 150,000 cardiovascular events. They found that as LDL increases independent of all other blood markers or risk factors, there was a remarkably consistent dose-dependent relationship with cardiovascular disease and concluded that 'LDL unequivocally causes atherosclerotic cardiovascular disease'.

cancer, compared to those following higher-carb diets.[15] A major reason for these health effects was not so much the absence of carbohydrates per se, but the food choices that were used to replace those calories. These typically appear to have included animal foods high in saturated fats such as red meat and butter, combined with a lack of foods rich in polyphenols and fibre such as vegetables, fruits and whole grains. That's not to say it's *impossible* to have a 'healthy keto' style diet. Hypothetically, if you were to consume lots of high-fibre, low-carb vegetables and unsaturated fats from nuts, seeds and fatty fish in place of red meat, that would likely counteract many of the associated health risks.

The bottom line: The ketogenic diet can be a reasonable short-term strategy for weight loss, management of type 2 diabetes and other metabolic derangements. However, there are consistent downsides related to continued adherence – notably its impact on liver and cardiometabolic health – which mean it is typically not an optimal diet for long-term health.

Diet myth no. 2: Intermittent fasting is just calorie restriction

Intermittent fasting (IF) is an eating pattern where a person alternates between periods of fasting and eating. There are many variations of IF, including alternate-day fasting (ADF) and intermittent energy restriction, where you consume, say, 25 per cent of your normal calorie allowance on three days of the week. However, people will probably be most familiar with the 16:8 or 20:4 methods, which dictate how long you fast for per day (i.e. 16 or 20 hours of fasting, and either 8 or 4 hours of eating).

The premise is that, as ancient hunter-gatherers, we would often go through long periods when food was scarce; and as a result, our bodies are very well adapted to coping with fasting. Common claims for IF's benefits include the body slowing down into 'repair mode' and turning on something called autophagy, which acts to clear out damaged cells and induces life-preserving changes. There is also the idea that fasting keeps insulin levels to a minimum, which allows the body time to burn fat.

According to a survey by the International Food Information Council, IF has become the most popular diet in America, with multiple studies supporting its efficacy for weight loss. As the popularity of IF grows, new methods and subtypes arise, creating even more unanswered questions. However, despite numerous variations arising, it appears that the vast majority of the benefits of IF are simply attributable to the calorie deficit imposed.*[16]

It is worth mentioning that in a few specific scenarios, however, IF does appear to be superior to a simple caloric restriction wherein a person eats fewer calories but at whatever time of day they like. To preface the chrononutrition chapter later, which is about the science of meal timing, the first scenario to consider is when a person allocates their eating window to the earlier part of the day – also called early time-restricted feeding (eTRF). The most rigorous and controlled feeding trial on this topic was completed in 2018. Eight men with pre-diabetes underwent a five-week study in which all meals were provided, and this was designed to keep subjects the same weight. The meals had to be eaten under supervision at prescribed times.[17] Each man was randomized a six-hour feeding window that ended before 3 p.m., or a twelve-hour feeding window that included eating late into the evening (which represents most people). The study found that those who stopped eating at 3 p.m. had improved insulin sensitivity, beta-cell

* This brand-new meta-analysis on twenty-seven RCTs tested different intermittent fasting protocols such as 16:8, 20:4, and even alternate-day and 5:2 fasting with each other, and pitted them against normal calorie restriction. Researchers found no differences in weight loss, insulin sensitivity and various blood lipids. Similar results from other analyses found no differences apart from IF leading to a greater reduction in waist circumference.

responsiveness (the cells within the pancreas that are responsible for releasing insulin), blood pressure, oxidative stress and a reduced appetite. These results suggest that confining your meals to the earlier part of the day may aid in blood glucose regulation, cardiovascular health and weight management. What makes this study revolutionary is that it was the first study *ever* to demonstrate that eTRF improves aspects of cardiometabolic health independent of weight loss. These findings have been solidified by many free-living studies cited in the chrononutrition chapter (see page 101). So, it appears that IF can have inherent benefits for aspects of cardiometabolic health when the eating window is confined to the earlier part of the day.

Another promising field of intermittent fasting research that is slowly emerging is the concept of autophagy and how it relates to cancer. It might help here to imagine our bodies as a bustling city, where everyday waste and old buildings regularly need to be cleared away for new construction. This is similar to the process of autophagy. It's like our internal recycling and garbage disposal system, breaking down old, damaged cells and creating new, healthy ones. Autophagy helps keep our bodies running smoothly, just as a clean city is more efficient and pleasant to live in.[18]

Scientists have observed that activities like sleeping, exercising, and eating fewer calories can rev up the process of autophagy, but fasting might have its own unique way of turning up the dial. Studies in rodents have shown that fasting for more than twenty-four hours can reduce levels of a molecule called insulin-like growth factor-1 (IGF-1).[19] This is interesting because lowering IGF-1 appears to encourage the body to make more stem cells, which could potentially be helpful in managing cancer. Regular calorie restriction, without fasting, doesn't seem to have the same impact on IGF-1 unless protein is also reduced in the diet.[20] There's some early evidence in humans that prolonged fasting might make chemotherapy less toxic and slow tumour growth in certain cancer patients,[21] although importantly the evidence isn't yet strong enough to make a broad recommendation. There are currently several large studies happening that are investigating this further, though, so we'll need to stay tuned for those results.

Nonetheless, it's important to remember that fasting, especially for extended periods, isn't without its risks. In particular, prolonged fasting can lead to cachexia, which is like a severe drought that causes the dangerous wasting away of muscle and fat. For cancer patients in particular, getting enough nutrition is crucial. In fact, about one-third of cancer patients die due to heart or lung failure as a result of cachexia, which is why extended fasts should only be done if your healthcare team gives you the green light.

In short, the connection between intermittent fasting, autophagy and cancer is an important area of research that's unfolding. As we wait for more results, it's essential to remember that any changes to diet, especially in the context of a disease like cancer, should be guided by healthcare professionals.

The bottom line: Intermittent fasting is a perfectly viable strategy to aid weight loss and the management of type 2 diabetes and other metabolic diseases. The majority of IF's benefits are largely down to simple caloric restriction – however, there are some scenarios in which IF appears superior to regular dieting. These include eTRF being more beneficial for metabolic health, appetite and weight loss, as well as evidence suggesting benefits for prolonged fasts in specific cancer-treatment protocols. That being said, engaging in IF has been associated with greater eating-disorder symptomology, so if you struggle with hard 'food rules' then it likely isn't advisable for you.[22]

Diet myth no. 3: A vegan diet is always healthy

Walk into any plant-based café or restaurant these days and you're inundated with a vast range of options, from vegan mac 'n' cheese and 'bleeding' beetroot burgers, to vegetable katsu curry and Kentucky fried chick'n. Veganism no longer means a dry, sad bowl of lifeless lettuce leaves, soggy tofu and a few unseasoned edamame beans.

One in five people in the UK now identifies as vegan, and plant-based alternatives are becoming ever more popular. The vegan food industry is valued at over $26.8 billion, and is set to surpass $65 billion by 2030.[23] Even those who aren't prepared to give up their steak or breakfast bacon any time soon are reducing their intake of animal products, with a third of British consumers now having regular 'meat-free' days, and almost one in three of us regularly buying plant 'milks' (even though plants don't lactate). Widespread movements and initiatives such as Veganuary in the UK have led many major brands, such as KFC, McDonald's, Greggs and Pizza Hut, to offer vegan alternatives. The argument goes that eating a plant-based diet will stop animal suffering, save the environment, improve our health and add years onto our life expectancy. But is veganism really the holy grail for us and the planet?

As with those who follow keto diets, vegans typically have lower BMIs and a reduced risk of heart disease and type 2 diabetes. A large component of these benefits is simply due to plant foods being less calorically dense, with greater levels of fibre and micronutrients, thus making it harder to overeat and become overweight. Many studies have also looked at the effects of a plant-based diet on health and longevity, but this is heavily context dependent. A meta-analysis of forty observational studies including over 190,000 people found that vegans consume less saturated fat and have lower BMIs, waist circumference, LDL, blood pressure and blood glucose compared to their omnivorous counterparts.[24] This is why other analyses of multiple studies have shown vegans have a 10 per cent reduced risk of cardiovascular disease.[25]

However, 'unhealthful' plant-based diets, which are rich in

refined grains, potatoes, sweets and added sugars – and which contain lower levels of fibre, unsaturated fats and antioxidants – lead to an increased risk of cardiovascular disease. In the analysis of several large studies from Taiwan, the vegan diet was not found to be superior for cardiometabolic blood markers compared to the meat-eating controls. This may have been related to the fact that the staple Taiwanese diet is rich in rice, vegetables such as broccoli, asparagus and carrots, and noodles and soups, as well as seafood and meat.

Context matters. If you're switching to a vegan diet from a standard Western diet that is full of ultra-processed snacks, fried meats and hyper-palatable and overly sugary pastries, then of course you'll improve your health and feel much better – even if your vegan diet isn't picture-perfect. The inevitable increase in vegetables, fruits, legumes and grains will do wonders for your overall health, although your gut might struggle to begin with (we'll talk more about that in the gut microbiome chapter). But when you compare the diets of a 'healthful' vegan to a healthful omnivore following something like the Mediterranean diet (MD) in a controlled setting, then the results aren't as glaringly obvious.

In one study, twenty-four healthy young adults followed a four-week vegan or Mediterranean-style diet *ad libitum* (which means they ate until they were satisfied).[26] Both groups made dietary changes that led to reductions in saturated fat and increases in fibre. While those on the vegan diet reduced their cholesterol and body weight to a greater extent, the Mediterranean diet was stronger in improving microvascular function (blood vessel health). This is probably due to relative increases in polyphenols, as they are found in olive oil, and vegetables rich in nitrates, such as leafy green veg and beetroot, which vasodilate (widen) our vessels. Similarly, researchers concluded that while both diets may offer cardiovascular risk-reduction benefits, the MD appears to be superior in this respect, due to improvements in vasodilatory ability.

The twelve-week CARDIVEG (Cardiovascular Prevention with Vegetarian Diet) Study was similarly balanced in its findings, comparing the MD to a lacto-ovo vegetarian diet. While both reduced body weight and fat mass, the vegetarian diet was more effective in lowering LDL, whereas the MD led to a greater reduction in triglyceride levels.[27]

Truthfully, almost any dietary pattern can be done well or poorly (excluding ones that restrict multiple food groups, such as the carnivore diet). A vegan diet that prioritizes health will be low in ultra-processed low-fibre plant substitutes, while emphasizing whole grains, fruits and veggies, and adequate amounts of protein from soybeans, tempeh, edamame and wheat-based proteins. It will also prioritize a healthy amount of unsaturated fatty acids from beans, nuts, oils and seeds.

Vegan diet considerations

There are a few areas in which vegans need to be particularly mindful about their dietary choices. One is the increased risk of nutrient deficiencies in vitamin B12 and iron, which are typically found in greater concentrations in animal products and are harder to come by in plants and grains. Vitamin B12 deficiency (characterized by tiredness, mood swings and tingling in the arms and legs) is common among vegans, and the risk is especially high if you don't take a B12 supplement.[28] Iron is essential to make haemoglobin, which carries oxygen around the body, and vegans tend to have lower iron stores and a higher prevalence of iron-deficiency anaemia.[29] This is because the iron found in legumes, leafy greens and nuts (non-heme iron) isn't very bioavailable (only 1–10 per cent is absorbed).[30] As such, people who follow a vegan diet need 1.8 times the recommended daily intake (RDI) compared to those who eat meat. Plant foods loaded with iron include red kidney beans, which have around 6mg per cooked cup (35 per cent RDI), and 6oz of tofu provides 2.5mg (14 per cent RDI).

Perhaps a bigger concern is the rise in veganism among children. While it is possible to have healthy vegan children, it isn't easy and there are serious consequences if you get it wrong. Studies have shown that children raised on a vegan diet are often smaller and have low levels of certain nutrients such as riboflavin and B12. Extreme instances of such deficiencies have led to high-profile deaths.[31] Some countries, such as France, have passed laws stating that raising a child as a vegan is criminal neglect and that all school meals must contain both meat and animal products. As veganism becomes more popular in adolescents, emerging evidence suggests that about 50 per cent of patients with anorexia nervosa have tried some form of vegetarian- or vegan-style dieting.[32] Psychologically, it's been suggested that a vegan lifestyle could further simplify the lives of people with an eating pathology in terms of providing clear dos and don'ts, which may allow worsening mental restrictions to arise under the guise of 'choosing' to be vegan.[33]

The bottom line: The vegan diet can be done extremely well if packed with minimally processed, whole plant foods, but it is essential to watch out for certain issues. Make sure to consume lots of B12-fortified foods such as plant milks, breakfast cereals, spreads and soy products, and take a B12 supplement just in case. Iron-rich foods include fortified cereals, beans, lentils, cashew nuts and chia seeds. If you're aware that your relationship with food isn't ideal, or that your health anxiety overburdens you at times, it probably isn't wise to follow a vegan diet.

Diet myth no. 4: Animal protein is better than plant protein

Protein quality often comes up in debates between the vegan and omnivorous crowds, especially in the fitness community. The belief that animal proteins are simply superior is an all too controversial and emotional topic for many. People argue that proteins derived from animal sources such as meat, fish, eggs and whey (dairy) are 'complete' proteins, as they contain all nine essential amino acids in adequate amounts, whereas only a handful of plant-based proteins – such as soybeans, peas and quinoa – come close. In addition, plant-based sources contain fibres that impede the access of enzymes to proteins and can induce a decrease in protein digestibility.[34] The major difference between animal proteins and plant proteins, however, is that the nutrient leucine is available in significantly higher quantities in animal proteins.

Leucine is the most important amino acid for muscle building, and it is largely responsible for stimulating muscle protein synthesis (muscle-building response).[35] The other concern among the fitness community is that plant proteins aren't as protein-dense per calorie compared to animal proteins – meaning in order for hefty 'gym bros' to reach their 200g protein intake for the day, for instance, they'd need to chomp down six entire blocks of tofu or eleven cups of lentils. Compare that to the much more manageable three medium-sized chicken breasts, two eggs and a pint of milk for an omnivore.

This all being said, when studies directly compare a high-protein plant-based diet (>1.6g/kg) with an omnivorous diet, there don't appear to be significant differences in muscle growth or strength.[36] However, it should be highlighted that these studies are short-term, and because building muscle is a long-term process, finding statistical differences over the short-term proves to be difficult, therefore, we don't know for sure that a high-protein plant-based diet leads to similar muscle-growth outcomes over the long term.

When it comes to the nutritional quality of animal and vegan proteins, there are other aspects to consider, too. While there are notable differences between the absorption rates of plant and animal proteins, these are likely to be negligible providing you eat enough protein overall. What 'enough' means we don't really know, but generally, the higher the better. To assess how much of a nutrient we can access in a particular food, we use bioavailability data. This is based on scoring scales such as the Digestible Indispensable Amino Acid Score (DIAAS), which assesses the digestibility and absorbability of feeding raw plant proteins to pigs.[37] While human digestive tracts are much more similar to those of pigs than of rats, ultimately we aren't pigs (well, most of us aren't, anyway) and so it isn't an exact science.

When we assess properly prepared plant proteins in humans, where you soak, sprout or cook them prior to consumption, the differences in bioavailability compared to animal proteins are much smaller. We need to also acknowledge the nutritional differences between these foods. For example, lentils are rich in unsaturated fats, phytonutrients and fibre, all of which are extremely health-promoting, compared to a rib-eye steak which, although much more protein-dense, is rich in saturated fat and low in fibre. When we discuss protein quality, we should consider the effect that protein-rich foods have on overall health, not just their ability to grow your bicep an inch. On the other hand, in the context of an elderly population who don't eat enough protein due to a declining appetite, and who may have poor accessibility to different foods due to geographical location or low income, then lean animal proteins low in saturated fats are likely superior for general health and for muscle retention.

The bottom line: If you have adequate access to food, sufficient income and are able to eat a sufficient amount of protein from a mixture of plant-based foods (>1.6g/kg), then there probably isn't a big difference in muscle-building properties between plant-based and animal proteins. That being said, with the exception of fatty fish and low-fat dairy products, minimally processed plant-based proteins are typically more health-promoting than animal proteins.

Diet myth no. 5: Producing meat is not harmful to the environment

Many people choose veganism because of environmental concerns. Unsustainable deforestation for agriculture, which cuts down up to 15 billion trees annually, is the main cause of biodiversity loss globally. This threatens our climate, as forests not only regulate rainfall and maintain soil quality, but also absorb carbon dioxide. Disturbing this system means stored greenhouse gases are released, contributing to about 10 per cent of global warming. Halting deforestation is key to addressing the climate crisis.

Among various agricultural practices, the meat and dairy industries are the most detrimental, due to the significant pollution, greenhouse gas emissions and consumption of fossil fuels, water and land which they require. Half of all habitable land worldwide is used for agriculture, primarily to raise livestock or grow their feed, which results in a large carbon footprint. Research indicates that transitioning to a plant-based diet could reduce the land required for agriculture by 75 per cent, freeing up space equivalent to all of North America and Brazil combined.[38]

Even without adopting a fully vegan diet, reducing our intake of red meat and dairy could substantially decrease agricultural land use, as this would lessen the need for pastures and crop farming. The reason is the inefficiency of energy transfer from plants to animals and then to humans. For instance, beef has an energy efficiency of only 2 per cent, meaning that only 2kcal of beef is produced for every 100kcal fed to a cow.[39] Reducing red meat consumption can thus limit caloric loss and reduce the need for farmland, allowing for the restoration of natural vegetation and ecosystems.

But vegan diets aren't necessarily healthy, despite what many people think. Most of the benefits are attributable to eating a greater variety and number of plants and fibre sources, which should be a target for all healthful dietary patterns. As is the case with any diet, veganism can be done extremely healthily or poorly. With the introduction of ultra-processed vegan 'junk' foods, simply switching to a plant-based diet doesn't guarantee an improvement in health. An optimal dietary pattern should include a wide variety of plant-based foods, including whole grains, lots of fruits and veggies, adequate amounts of protein from soybeans, legumes, tempeh, edamame and wheat-based proteins, and a sufficient amount of unsaturated fatty acids from beans, nuts, oils and seeds. Regarding muscle gains, as long as you're consuming >1.6g/kg of protein a day from a variety of plant-based proteins, you don't need to concern yourself with missing out on *much* muscle. The intensity and progression of your workouts will always be more important regardless.

Even if you don't want to become vegan, consider reducing your consumption of meat and dairy to have a tremendously beneficial impact on the environment and global warming. If everyone (who is fortunate enough to be able to) started cutting out meat and dairy just one day a week, we would all reap the benefits in the long run.

The bottom line: Vegan diets aren't always healthy. They can be done very well or very poorly, depending on what plant-based foods you eat. However, they *are* always far more environmentally friendly. Reducing the amount of meat and increasing the amount of plant-based foods you eat (even only slightly) will have a beneficial impact in terms of sustainability.

Diet myth no. 6: The carnivore diet is healthy

The carnivore diet is a meat lover's dream. Burger patties, eggs, cheese and steak dripping in butter? *Sign me up!* you might be thinking. In this diet plan, you eat meat or animal products for every meal. Think of it as the ketogenic diet on steroids. But unlike keto, which limits carbs and plants to a low level, the carnivore diet excludes all plant foods including vegetables, fruits, grains, legumes, nuts and seeds.

Adherents claim the diet improves mental clarity, raises energy levels, improves gut health and boosts the treatment of auto-immune and chronic diseases. Its recent rise to fame is somewhat attributable to an orthopaedic surgeon named Shawn Baker, who released the book *The Carnivore Diet* in 2018. Unsurprisingly, it is full of appeals to 'ancestry arguments', along with anecdotes of people miraculously curing their ailments through following the diet.

Appealing to ancestry or tradition is a type of logical fallacy, arguing that a practice or belief is correct or superior simply because it has been done for a long time. The overriding theme regarding the carnivore diet is that we should eat like strong hunter-gatherers and cavemen once did. If only these people knew that meat wasn't the only thing we ate back then. The caveman diet in fact largely consisted of fruit, vegetables, leaves, flowers, bark, insects . . . and then *some* meat. I should probably mention that the New Mexico Medical Board revoked Baker's medical licence in 2017.

Toxic plants?

Carnivore zealots often state that plant foods are toxic, because certain vegetables contain compounds such as lectins and phytic acid (found in beans, legumes and whole grains, said to damage the gut) or isocyanates (found in cruciferous vegetables, which are said to damage the thyroid).

In the interest of your time and sanity, let's just debunk one of these so-called toxic compounds now. Phytic acid is typically referred to as an 'anti-nutrient' by proponents of the carnivore way, because it can decrease the absorption of minerals like iron and zinc.[40] But that's only one part of the story. Why leave out the fact that beans, for instance, contain a lot of zinc, and people who consume them aren't typically deficient in these minerals? Or that simply cooking or soaking pulses reduces phytic acid content by 80 per cent?[41] Not to mention that phytic acid actually has a lot of benefits. It reduces oxidative stress, serum cholesterol and renal stone formation, and decreases blood sugar responses by inhibiting the activity of amylase (an enzyme that breaks down carbohydrates into simple sugars).[42] If phytic acid really was a problem, we would expect to see evidence of increasing disease risk in foods rich in phytic acid. Yet a meta-analysis of twenty-three cohort studies and randomized controlled trials (RCTs) on beans and health outcomes showed an 11 per cent reduced risk of cardiovascular disease, a 22 per cent reduction in heart disease, and even evidence for slowing down the growth of certain cancer cells.[43] Beans might make you fart (if your gut isn't used to them, or you have IBS), but at least you'll be healthy while letting rip!

Toxic meat?

Ironically though, many compounds in meat can be considered 'toxic'. For instance, did you know there is a small amount of formaldehyde in beef? Formaldehyde is a poison . . . so obviously beef is bad for you, right? On a similar note, choline is an essential compound for various metabolic processes, which is found in red meat and liver, but when we break down choline in the gut, it produces secondary metabolites, or by-products, called trimethylamine N-oxide (TMAO). TMAO has been shown to increase the risk of primary liver cancer in both rats and humans.[44] Not to mention heme iron and heterocyclic amines (HCAs), with data showing these meat compounds have carcinogenic and atherosclerotic properties.[45]

Do you see how easy it is to pick a random compound in a food and claim it's harmful to us? What matters is the dose. If you were to extract phytic acid from seeds, nuts and legumes and eat a ludicrous amount of it, or extract heme iron from beef and concentrate it in a pill form, then yes, it would likely have negative effects. However, this is entirely illogical, as these compounds aren't consumed in isolation, and the foods in which they're consumed contain a myriad of different nutrients that all affect health differently. Not to mention that the dosages of the 'toxins' found in plants are so small that they don't have a harmful effect, they have a hormetic effect – the body beneficially adapts in response to a stressor.

There's also a habit many of us practise every single day that increases inflammation in the body, causes oxidative stress and cellular damage and increases our blood pressure.[46] It sounds bad, right? But I'm talking about exercise. Exercise is a stressor; but over time it causes the body to beneficially adapt to greatly benefit our heart, lungs, muscle, bone and brain. The same thing happens when you lift weights. Short-term damage, pain and inflammation occur from squatting heavy weights, but over the long term it leads to greater functionality, muscle size, strength and bone health. Similarly, it is thought that playing around in the dirt as a child allows the body to build immunity and reduces the risk of auto-immune and allergic diseases – termed the 'hygiene hypothesis'.[47]

Moreover, plant 'toxins' aren't even toxic, as the definition for a toxin (a poisonous substance) requires that it be harmful to the body at the dosages in question, which is absolutely not the case for the dosages found in food. Indeed, all the human evidence on plant foods and health outcomes, demonstrated in a study of ninety-six systematic reviews, shows that fruit and vegetables are overwhelmingly health-promoting, and substantially reduce the risk of cardiovascular disease, diabetes, liver disease, cancer, bone diseases and death from all causes.[48]

A Big Mis-STEAK

The potential negatives of the carnivore diet are alarming. As we've already seen in relation to the keto diet, excluding all plant foods while consuming an abundance of red meat and saturated fat is a terrible idea for your health. Evidence from over 171 research studies found that consuming more than 50g of red meat per day increases your risk of colon cancer by 21 per cent.[49] The amounts that red meat is consumed in a carnivore-style diet would far exceed this threshold, rendering the true increase in cancer risk unknown. Not to mention that when saturated fat intake exceeds 10 per cent of total energy (roughly 25–30g), the direct increase in cardiovascular disease events is huge! This is demonstrated in a meta-analysis of fifteen controlled human trials showing that reducing saturated-fat intake reduces combined cardiovascular disease events by 21 per cent.[50]

One anecdote demonstrates this perfectly: Michael Reilly (who goes by the handle @TheCarnivoreKid on Twitter) was a young man with a family, feeling on top of the world. He had washboard abs, and enjoyed cardio training and lifting weights five times a week. In December 2021, though, he was found to have three blocked arteries and heart disease, and he suffered a stroke.

How did this come about? He had been on a low-carb carnivore-style diet since 2016, with an LDL cholesterol of >190mg/dL. Fortunately, triple-artery bypass surgery saved his life. If you're considering the carnivore diet, remember Michael's story. You can't 'feel' LDL particles in your arteries building up plaque. You can't 'feel' carcinogenic processes occurring in your gut. You can't 'feel' systemic inflammation creeping up on you and damaging cells throughout the body. These things spring up on you, and before you know it, it's too late.

The bottom line: The carnivore diet is an extremely restrictive and unhealthy dietary pattern. The mechanistic basis which advocates rely on largely stems from animal or cell-culture studies, yet they choose to ignore the irresistible amount of human evidence showing that the consumption of plants improves health. Long-term data illustrating the health risks of the carnivore diet will likely be published in the next ten or so years, and as it is even more restrictive than the keto diet, I can't believe the prognosis will be good. Until then, don't bet your life on it. It's not worth it.

Diet myth no. 7: The Mediterranean diet is overhyped

When we think of a 'diet' these days, we usually think of some kind of restriction that will help us reach a specific outcome, such as weight loss. The Mediterranean diet (MD) couldn't be further from that. Rather, it encourages an eating pattern that includes the food staples of people from countries surrounding the Mediterranean Sea, such as Greece, Spain, Italy and France. One important aspect of this way of eating that is often forgotten is the focus on community. Think of wide table spreads with family and friends laughing and sharing food; this sort of eating does wonders for your psychological health, and goes a long way to helping your physical health, too. It's not just the food we consume, but the social situation impacting our psychology which has an overall positive effect on our health.

The key principle of the MD emphasizes a majority plant-based eating approach:

- A diet loaded with vegetables, fruits, whole grains, legumes, nuts and seeds, which are minimally processed.
- Olive oil as the principal source of fat.
- Cheese and yoghurt, consumed daily in low to moderate amounts.
- Fish and poultry, consumed in low to moderate amounts a few times a week.
- Red meat consumed infrequently and in small amounts.

Eating this way leaves little room for processed fare. When you look at a plate of food it should be bursting with colour and contain a variety of different foods.

The MD has repeatedly demonstrated heart-healthy results in

both observational and controlled studies. One meta-analysis of forty-one studies showed that those who most adhere to the MD had a 21–38 per cent lower risk of cardiovascular disease versus those adhering the least.[51] It's also been shown to be effective at helping people lose weight, which is largely attributable to its emphasis on minimally processed, nutritious foods and on all foods in moderation.[52]

However, this way of eating can become expensive and is not always an option for everyone. Many people are forced to buy 'processed' foods or ready meals due to food insecurity, the cost-of-living crisis, the lack of healthful food policy by governments to keep unprocessed foods more affordable, and a lack of accessibility or time. But remember one thing: just because you consume processed foods, that doesn't automatically mean you're destined for poor health. Many affordable, commonly demonized processed foods are great for you, including canned beans, protein powders, soy milk, frozen vegetables, nut butters, tofu, canned fish, hummus, rotisserie chicken, pre-cooked rice, and lentil and pasta packs.

The bottom line: There's very little negative to say about the MD apart from its potential to be expensive. It's a fantastic health-promoting dietary pattern and encompasses most of the dietary principles for preventative health we discuss in this book.

Diet myth no. 8: Your blood type matters when it comes to dieting

The year 1996 saw a popular book published that claimed people can become healthier, live longer and achieve their ideal weight by eating according to their blood type. It argued that a person's choice of condiments, spices and even exercise should all depend on their blood type. The book was a bestseller and led to a rush of people researching their blood type, revising their grocery lists and changing how they ate.

The book's claims included that people with type O blood should eat seafood, broccoli and red meat and perform high-intensity aerobic exercise to lose weight, while those with type A should consume vegetables, pineapple, olive oil and soy to achieve the same effect. Let's just end this here and now. A systematic review in 2013 scoured the depths of medical journals to find any evidence for the efficacy of this diet and came up with . . . nothing.[53] More recently, studies in the last ten years show that adherence to the blood-type diet can improve certain health markers, but those benefits are completely unrelated to any one individual's blood type.

The bottom line: While some of the suggestions within blood-type dieting (like eating more broccoli) could improve your health, that has absolutely nothing to do with your blood type. As with many popular diets, it's just another made-up, unsubstantiated hypothesis easily dismissed by real evidence.[54]

Diet myth no. 9: Alkaline foods are better than acidic ones

The alkaline diet is centred on the theory that the root cause of disease is excess acidity in the body. Therefore, to treat and cure disease (including, supposedly, even cancer), 'acid-forming foods' like meat, fish and lentils should be avoided and replaced with 'alkaline-forming foods' like fruit and vegetables. Robert Oldham Young is widely regarded as the founder of this diet, having published several books on the topic – including *The pH Miracle*, which sold millions of copies. He claims that, on digesting food, you produce either acidotic or alkalotic by-products, which influence disease and cancer risk.

However, it's practically impossible for diet to impact blood pH, because of acid-base homeostasis. It's crucial for our blood to remain within a very narrow pH range (7.35–7.45);[55] if our blood falls out of this range, it can be fatal, as in diabetic ketoacidosis or heart arrhythmias from alkalosis. This is why our body regulates blood pH through mechanisms such as: breathing out CO_2 (acidic), kidneys producing bicarbonate (alkalotic), or excreting acid through urine. As such, food literally cannot change our blood pH.

A systematic review in 2016 found one study on the alkaline diet, and unsurprisingly concluded that there is no evidence to support it.[56] There's recent evidence showing that the dietary acid load could slightly affect bone mineral density, but this depends on how the acid load is measured.[57] This is likely due to a difference in the nutritional components of food and not its 'acidity'. Oh, and it's probably a good idea to tell you that, in 2017, Mr Young was convicted for illegally practising medicine on people at his ranch, without a licence.

The bottom line: If you are considering rejecting evidence-based medical therapies in favour of the alkaline diet as a treatment for cancer (or any other disease), just don't. While there is some evidence that certain diets can slow the progression of cancer, or work as a supervised adjuvant treatment with chemotherapy, *diet cannot cure cancer*. Many people could benefit from increasing their fruit and vegetable intake, but that has nothing to do with alkalinity.

Diet myth no. 10: Detox diets can be trusted

Before it was co-opted in the recent wellness craze, the word 'detox' was reserved for a medical treatment to rid the body of dangerous, often life-threatening levels of alcohol, drugs or poisons. I can recall several of my patients coming into hospital hallucinating as a result of various concoctions of street drugs and unknown substances they had injected into their bodies. These patients would undergo medical detoxification, which involves specialized drugs and therapies to help protect the body while it attempts to flush out the harmful compounds. One product we give to patients who have overdosed is activated charcoal – it binds to toxins in the stomach, preventing their absorption.[58]

The detox protocols now being championed by the wellness industry come in all shapes and sizes, including juice cleanses, supplement pills, detox teas, and heavy metal and even parasite cleanses. The millennial need to detox seems to be born out of our obsession with purity and the guilt we feel for living a fast-paced, sometimes hedonistic lifestyle that makes us feel tired and drained. The concept that a few drops of liquid detox can fix years of stress, alcohol, poor sleep and living life at 100 miles an hour is very appealing, for sure. This narrative promotes the idea that our environment or lifestyle is 'toxic', and that we need to manually cleanse ourselves to be healthy. It's appealing because it plays on people's desires to find a quick fix for everything, as opposed to focusing on the lifestyle changes necessary to see a meaningful difference in the long term.

I'm not for one second suggesting that we can't support our bodies in the detoxification process by eating well and exercising. However, the human body has many sophisticated mechanisms by which it detoxes itself, and these mechanisms are far smarter than any solution you can conjure up. Your liver, kidneys, bowel, skin and lungs all play an essential role in detoxification.[59]

Importantly, almost all the claims made by companies and advocates selling 'detox' products are entirely unsubstantiated. No, they won't cure your autoimmune disease, depression, autism or ADHD (ironically, their phrasing unhelpfully stigmatizes people living with these conditions, labelling them as 'impure' or 'toxic'). No, they won't fix your skin or gut issues. Although there is some evidence that 'heavy metal detox' products can remove some minerals from your body, they don't distinguish between essential and non-essential minerals, and they've been shown to diminish levels of sodium and calcium.[60]

Finally, even if some unwanted minerals were extracted, there is no evidence that this process effectively treats any medical condition or presentation.

The bottom line: Any manifestation of a 'detox' diet or product is likely unregulated if not an outright scam, and potentially very dangerous. The body is well equipped to dispose of potentially harmful compounds by itself, and in cases where toxins can cause illness (e.g. high levels of asbestos exposure from construction work), that cannot be undone by a pill or juice cleanse. Focusing on the lifestyle principles in this book is the best way to aid your body in its detoxification process.

Diet myth no. 11: Tons of protein is needed to gain muscle

For those who are training towards exercise or strength goals, there is a lot of confusion and misinformation about how, what and when to eat around your training in order to optimize performance in the gym and make those coveted gains in muscle.

First, let me make one thing clear: you can eat as much protein as you like, as often as you like, but if you're not working out in the gym at the right intensity and volume, you'll reach a growth limit very quickly. Second, the amount of protein you require to grow will depend on the situation, the stakes (i.e. are you a recreational athlete or a high-stakes competitor?) and your goal.

Importantly, the recommended daily allowance for protein of 0.8g/kg is only the bare minimum to prevent adverse health effects from protein deficiencies (brittle nails and hair, poor fluid balance, weakness, fatigue, diarrhoea). It is not the 'optimal amount' for health. When we hit 1.2–1.6g/kg a day, this should be enough for the majority of people seeking to optimize their health.[61] When thinking about muscle building and exercise performance specifically, though, if consuming a diet with adequate energy (i.e. eating at maintenance or above, which means that you're eating at least as many calories as you burn) then 1.6g/kg is really the sweet spot. Going above this to 1.6–2.2g/kg is perfectly fine, but it follows the law of diminishing returns; you'll only get minor benefits.[62]

For an adult weighing 80kg, consuming 1.6g/kg would equate to 128g of protein. In real food terms, that's the equivalent of two chicken breasts and a pint of milk. For the vegans out there, we're talking a soy protein drink, a block of tofu, a cup of lentils and some oats. Now, if you're actively dieting, losing weight or are an advanced athlete (often defined as having consistently trained for >5 years), then some evidence suggests that going above 2.2g/kg (>1g/lb) of protein per day will preserve lean body mass to a greater extent and optimize athletic goals.[63]

Do we need to spread our protein intake out every few hours? Short answer: no. While there is evidence by world-leading exercise researcher Brad Schoenfeld suggesting that in order to maximize muscle hypertrophy (growth), one should consume protein at a target intake of 0.4g/kg per meal across a minimum of four meals in the day,[64] this conclusion is based on research strictly done on fast-digesting proteins in the absence of other macronutrients, whereas people don't eat meals like that. What the majority of us do (or should do at least) is consume balanced meals with fats, fibre, protein and carbs – which will slow down digestion, meaning a steady release of protein over time. Total protein intake in the day is by far the key driver of muscle growth, therefore as long as your meals are balanced, 2–3 high-protein meals a day should be sufficient.

The bottom line: For optimal health, consuming 1.2g–1.6g/kg of protein per day across at least two meals is ideal. If you're trying to put on muscle and are training consistently, then 1.6–2.2g/kg of protein per day will ensure you grow at the maximum rate. However, if you're actively losing weight, or are an advanced athlete with many years of training experience, then going above 2.2g/kg of protein per day may be wise to optimize progress.

Key takeaways

1. **No diet is going to be useful unless you can adhere to it.** In fact, all mainstream diets appear to have similar adherence rates on average,[65] which means your eating pattern should be highly individualized to what suits your dietary preferences and lifestyle.

2. **Any diet (whether it's covered in this book or not) can induce weight loss** through the same mechanism: by reducing total calorie intake and optimizing calorie expenditure, also called a calorie deficit. When calories and protein are matched, the diet you choose makes little difference to overall weight loss.

3. **Overly restrictive diets that eliminate entire food groups (e.g. keto and carnivore) can have dire consequences** that often go unnoticed for years, until it's too late. This can also apply to vegan diets if you're not sensible with your food choices. I'd strongly recommend against following a dietary pattern that outright excludes any food groups.

4. **The benefits of intermittent fasting are largely down to caloric restriction**, but there is growing evidence that earlier time-restricted feeding provides superior cardiometabolic benefits compared to eating across the day, independent of weight loss. There are other promising fields of research which demonstrate certain time-restricted feeding protocols may provide additional benefits beyond the ability to aid caloric restriction. Even if you don't fast intermittently, consuming most of your calories earlier in the day seems to be preferable.

5. **The vegan diet can improve many aspects of health if done sensibly, diversely and with adequate planning.**

The environmental impacts of animal agriculture are astonishing, and whether you want to be vegan or not, we should all consider reducing our red meat intake and increasing our plant consumption.

6. **Detoxes, the alkaline diet, blood-type diets and any other ridiculous fads you can think of are garbage and not rooted in science.** If you want a healthful dietary pattern, look no further than the Mediterranean diet.

7. **For optimal exercise performance and muscle building, aim for more than 1.6g/kg of protein per day, ideally consumed across at least two meals.** If you're super-advanced or attempting to 'cut', then going above 2.2g/kg is superior for retaining muscle. If you train in the morning, a high-carb meal 90–120 minutes prior to a workout can positively impact exercise performance, but post-workout carbs will not lead to greater hypertrophy or recovery unless you're due another intense session the same day.

PART TWO
Setting the Record Straight

In this section of the book, we will be debunking myths and tackling some of the most controversial topics in health and nutrition science. These include inflammation, weight as an indicator of health and the science of weight loss. So, lock in and look forward to having your previously held beliefs flipped on their head.

Inflammation

From Fork to Flame

Scroll online or visit a bookshop, and before long you'll see that inflammation has really become a buzzword. People are selling 'anti-inflammatory' diets anywhere and everywhere. They're dishing out recipes which (apparently) target specific illnesses, from inflammatory bowel disease through to arthritis and various other autoimmune diseases. And yet many of these marketers don't even understand what inflammation is.

Inflammation – it sounds intimidating, doesn't it? This biological response is often misunderstood and vilified, yet it is crucial for our survival, playing a vital role in healing injuries and combating infections. But what happens when this helpful ally turns into a relentless foe, inciting chronic health problems – and what role does our diet play in that transformation? This chapter will guide you through a vast landscape, where foods can either ignite the fires of inflammation or dampen their (sometimes) destructive flames. We'll start with busting some common myths on the subject, before delving deeper into the science behind pro-inflammatory and anti-inflammatory foods – arming you to make informed dietary decisions.

From the world's love affair with sugar to the fierce debate over omega-6 fats, from the misunderstood role of dairy to the surprising power of colourful berries and dark leafy greens, we will dissect the fact from the fiction. So, fasten your seat belts and prepare for an exciting exploration of how what we eat can influence inflammation – for better and for worse.

Inflammation myth no. 1: Seed oils are bad for you

Canola oil, vegetable oil, omega-6! How scary! Since hating on omega-6 fatty acids unfortunately became a thing, various people have harped on about how terrible these seed oils (the umbrella term for many plant-based oils) are, claiming they are highly inflammatory or cause heart disease because they're rich in omega-6s. One common misguided view is 'Seed oil consumption and obesity rates in the US are rising at the same time, so seed oils are the problem!' Okay, well, the number of people who drown by falling into a swimming pool actually correlates with the number of movies Nicolas Cage appears in on a yearly basis. Clearly Nicolas Cage is the reason for these deaths! But anyway, I digress.

It's easy to formulate a pseudoscientific case against omega-6 fats or polyunsaturated fatty acids (PUFAs). All you have to do is reference a couple of rodent studies from fifty years ago (not revealing to your audience that they were conducted on rats, of course), use glittery chemical language and sprinkle over the usual conspiratorial thinking that our ancestors supposedly thrived on saturated fats and nothing else. But closer inspection begins to illuminate the collection of standalone, unsubstantiated claims upon which their argument rests. Let's get into it.

The omega-6 inflammation scare is based on the hypothesis that the body converts the most common omega-6 fatty acid, linoleic acid, into another type of fatty acid called arachidonic acid. The latter has been implicated in increasing the number of pro-inflammatory cytokines in the body. However, this conversion process has only been demonstrated in animal studies and people have inappropriately attributed these effects to humans. The body doesn't convert *much* linoleic acid into arachidonic acid, because the process is highly inefficient. We have bucket loads of data showing that increasing levels of linoleic acid by over 500 per cent or decreasing levels by 90 per cent has no meaningful effect on arachidonic acid levels in the plasma, serum or red blood cells, all of which are within the blood.[1] And even in the small proportions that it could impact levels, arachidonic acid acts as both a pro- *and* anti-inflammatory mediator in many different inflammatory pathways.[2]

Now that we've ruined the fearmongers' entire mechanistic basis, let's look at real outcome data on the consumption of omega-6s and inflammation in the body. In studies conducted on actual *Homo sapiens*, not rodents, a high omega-6 intake doesn't seem to enhance inflammatory processes.[3] A recent meta-analysis of eighty-three controlled human studies (carried out by my university and former research-methods lecturer Lee Hooper, in fact) confirms this. They took various studies undertaken on people both with and without inflammatory bowel disease, and found that increasing omega-3, omega-6 or total polyunsaturated fatty acid intake had either little or no effect on inflammatory markers or risk of disease.[4]

But of course, seed oils aren't entirely composed of omega-6 fatty acids. The majority of them are actually monounsaturated fatty acids (MUFAs). So, let's leave omega-6 alone for a second and see whether cooking oils themselves are harmful to our health.

When all the major cooking oils were tested (including canola, peanut and corn oil), all were found to be more effective at reducing total and LDL (bad) cholesterol compared to butter or lard. This means that they are effective at reducing risk factors implicated in conditions such as heart disease and diabetes, especially when used as substitutes for other fats.[5] In fact, several studies demonstrated that vegetable oils can have an anti-inflammatory effect, with none of the ten human studies assessed showing an inflammatory response![6]

People often try to counter this by saying, 'But when you cook with them, they become oxidized, which causes inflammation.'

And yes, if you heat a seed oil up and keep it at a high enough temperature for a long time, like you would in deep-frying, you can absolutely cause the formation of trans-unsaturated fats. These are inherently damaging to our health, increase the risk of heart disease and death, and are indeed pro-inflammatory in nature.[7] However, in everyday cooking like pan-frying or roasting, this conversion process to trans fats just won't happen. You are not exposing the oil to high enough temperatures, nor are you cooking them for long enough for trans fats to form. For the vast majority of home cooking, it is not something to worry about.

And to close off one final point, what about the omega-3 to omega-6 ratio? Yes, it's also true that having higher tissue levels of omega-3 to omega-6 is beneficial (tissue levels meaning within fat, cell membranes, muscle, or organs like the heart and liver). However, there is little evidence to suggest that either serum levels or dietary levels have much of an influence on tissue levels.

The bottom line: Polyunsaturated fatty acids, omega-6s and seed oils are not inflammatory, nor is there strong evidence that they're a contributor to chronic disease. In fact, multiple studies in humans show they can even be anti-inflammatory! People who argue against this are hand-picking isolated, poorly designed research (mostly conducted on animals) and ignoring multiple lines of converging evidence from population-wide observational research, biomarker studies, metabolic wards and intervention studies in actual humans.

Inflammation myth no. 2: It's harmful to drink another mammal's milk

For many of us, dairy is a staple on our plate at every meal. But have you ever had a glass of milk or a large ice cream and felt your stomach cramping? Or have you noticed that you feel and look five months pregnant after just a few cheesy mozzarella bites? Well, I certainly have.

It's a commonly held belief that dairy causes inflammation. If people experience bloating, gas or a stomach upset, it's often automatically attributed to inflammation. And the line 'humans are the only species to drink another mammal's milk' is frequently used to imply that this is because our dairy consumption is unnatural and therefore bad. But remember, humans are also the only species to cook their food, drive cars, eat at restaurants and obtain information from social media. Should we stop doing all of that too?

Another reason people argue that dairy is inflammatory is because of the high saturated fat content. A large body of evidence has shown that saturated fat intake is positively associated with increased C-reactive protein (CRP) – the most robust indicator of inflammation in the body.[8] The 2020–25 American dietary guidelines recommend limiting saturated fat intake to less than 10 per cent of total calories per day. But hold the phone! Dairy also contains beneficial short-chain fatty acids and other nutrients that are strongly associated with heart and metabolic benefits. Doesn't that directly contradict what we know about saturated fats?

Before we dive in, it's important to understand that within 'dairy' is a complex range of individual foods, which vary a lot in terms of their form and processing. There are full-fat products and low-fat ones, where food manufacturers have mechanically separated the fat from liquid milk. You also have fermented products (kefir, yoghurt and cheese) where bioactive peptides may provide additional benefits for gut health and metabolic blood parameters (you can read more about this in the gut microbiome chapter).

You might be wondering which types of dairy (if any) you should include in your diet. Unfortunately, there is no simple answer. Some people (including myself) are unable to fully digest lactose, the sugar naturally present in milk products. If this is you,

you're probably all too familiar with the symptoms: gas, flatulence, bloating and diarrhoea. And even if you can digest lactose, you might be sensitive to other components of dairy products.* But back to saturated fats and dairy . . .

Since the 1960s, diets high in saturated fats have been linked to elevated LDL cholesterol levels and cardiovascular disease. More recently, research has cast doubts on what was previously seen as robust evidence. Inconsistent findings suggest that different types of saturated fats may have differing effects on blood lipids and heart health. A recent study published in the *International Journal of Cardiology* demonstrates this perfectly, in which scientists studied over 75,000 people from the UK and Denmark.[9]

Over a period of 13–18 years, close to 3,500 of these people had heart attacks. The scientists looked closely at the food habits and lifestyles of these people. They found that those who ate more shorter-carbon-chain fats (which are not found in meat) were less likely to have heart attacks. On the other hand, fats found in higher proportions in dairy products and plants, which have longer carbon chains, seemed to lower the risk of heart attacks. This study matches other research, which shows that the effect of fats from our food on our heart health can vary based on the length of the carbon chain.[10] While it's hard to say exactly which saturated fats are beneficial, there's consistent evidence that dairy saturated fats can be good for heart health.

There is also a role for the calcium in dairy to bind to fatty acids in the small intestine, forming 'calcium soaps' that prevent the absorption of those fats into the bloodstream.[11] In fact, a review of fifty-two studies found that dairy products can help reduce inflammation in people with conditions like diabetes or

---

* There has been some research into a specific type of dairy protein known as A1 beta-casein – found in most milk within the US. Research into this field is in its early stages and we're still learning about the other components of dairy and how they affect us.

heart disease.[12] Another analysis of eleven trials found that dairy products may improve inflammation indicators in adults.[13] This is important, because prolonged exposure to inflammation is often linked to heart disease and other health problems.

There are several proposed mechanisms by which dairy might suppress inflammatory pathways. One is that dairy contains high concentrations of an amino acid called leucine, which can increase adiponectin while decreasing oxidative stress. Adiponectin is an important fat-derived hormone that plays a vital role in protecting against insulin resistance and cardiovascular disease. This 'saviour hormone' binds to receptors and promotes a strong insulin-sensitizing effect (which improves our ability to regulate blood glucose), enhances fatty-acid oxidation and increases the number of mitochondria within a cell – as well as promoting anti-oxidative and anti-inflammatory effects.[14] Similarly, the protein sirtuin 1, which is also found in dairy, has been shown to increase the oxidative capacity of cells, thus preventing cellular damage.[15]

Still, even outside inflammation, many people are doubtful as to whether consuming dairy is beneficial for health. This should clear things up for you. A recent umbrella review looking at forty-one systematic reviews and meta-analyses, including hundreds of individual studies, analysed how milk consumption affected forty-five different health outcomes.[16] They found that for every 200ml of milk consumed per day, there was a 6 per cent reduced risk of cardiovascular disease, 7 per cent reduced risk of stroke, 4 per cent reduced risk of hypertension, 10 per cent reduced risk of colorectal cancer, 13 per cent reduced risk of metabolic syndrome, 39 per cent reduced risk of osteoporosis, and reduced risks of obesity, type 2 diabetes and Alzheimer's disease. They did, however, also find that milk consumption might be linked to higher rates of prostate cancer, Parkinson's disease and acne. Objectively speaking, this independent analysis highlights that the overwhelming amount of evidence shows that dairy is in fact health-promoting for the general population. And no, it wasn't funded by Big Milk (and even if it was, that's a poor reason to dismiss evidence – more information about this in the appendix).

The bottom line: Dairy has consistently been shown to have a neutral or even anti-inflammatory effect. Not all saturated fats are created equal, and the inflammatory potential of incorporating a variety of dairy products into your diet is not something to worry about. In fact, dairy may even benefit inflammation. It is also a quick and easy way to obtain lots of essential nutrients. However, if you do experience negative symptoms with dairy, you might want to trial lactose-free dairy options or consider an elimination diet. To do this, simply cut out all dairy for a few weeks while keeping other dietary habits constant, and check if your symptoms resolve. If you like, you can then try to slowly reintroduce dairy products over time, to see if you're able to tolerate them.

Inflammation myth no. 3: Sugar is always inflammatory

Don't put table sugar into your coffee! It causes inflammation! Or does it? In recent years, sugar has become public-health enemy number one. Previously, ingredients like fat and salt struck the most fear into the health-conscious, but over the last decade, a narrative has arisen presenting sugar as nothing but 'empty calories' which fill our plates and lead to diabetes and cancer. The public hysteria about sugar has influenced headlines touting it as 'more addictive than cocaine', and claiming it 'cooks you from the inside out' due to inflammation. This has led to millions of people 'quitting sugar' or replacing it with foods labelled as 'healthy' natural alternatives like coconut sugar or honey, which are often promoted by TikTokers and momfluencers. But what explains the rise of this sugar obsession? And is it true that there's more sugar in our diets than ever before?

Sugar is indeed added to many foods, and seems to be an

inescapable component of our modern diet. It's true that food manufacturers add sugar to products to enhance flavour, texture or as a preservative to increase shelf life. Many staple foods like bread, soups and sauces contain 'hidden' sugars for these exact reasons. Sugar is also naturally present in all carbohydrate-containing foods such as grains, fruits, vegetables and dairy. But is there a difference between natural and refined sugars? What does the science say about sugar's effect on inflammation?

An American study of forty-one overweight men and women increased their sugar consumption to 175g a day for ten weeks, of which more than 70 per cent was sugary drinks. At the end of the trial, the three key inflammatory markers (haptoglobin, CRP and transferrin) had increased by only 13, 5 and 6 per cent respectively – a tiny amount.[17] To put this into perspective, the equivalent of four cans of full sugar cola a day increased CRP from 1.8mg/L to 1.9mg/L, which is negligible. Only the increase in haptoglobin was statistically significant. The changes in CRP and transferrin were too small for the researchers to be confident they had even occurred. But doesn't this go against everything we've been told? Surely sugar is inflammatory? Let's look at some more research.

An analysis of thirteen studies addressed the effect that different dietary sugars (fructose, sucrose and glucose) have on biomarkers of subclinical inflammation.[18] The results were unremarkable. No differences were found between the fructose, glucose and sucrose groups, and total effects were only observed in a small number of studies, with the overall picture being inconsistent. These findings should stand out for one particular reason. If sugar was inherently inflammatory, we would have seen consistent increases in several inflammatory markers across different demographics and populations.

So, on the one hand we have many controlled trials showing that feeding people up to 200g of added sugar a day doesn't seem to significantly alter levels of circulating inflammatory biomarkers, while on the other hand, diets high in refined sugars score highly on the Dietary Inflammatory Index (see page 58), indicating a pro-inflammatory effect. What could explain this?

This in fact highlights a recognized issue in nutrition science. Translating the effect of a single nutrient on a single biomarker into an accurate reflection of the effect of a complex food matrix of other nutrients and overall dietary pattern on multifaceted processes like inflammation is often deceiving.

The ability of a food to affect bodily inflammation must be viewed through the lens of overall dietary habits, and not isolated foods or nutrients. This is why, in a controlled study where the only thing manipulated is the level of added sugar in the diet, consistent and statistically significant changes in inflammation aren't often observed. However, if you were to feed the intervention group the same food but increased their total calorie intake, replacing their fruit and vegetable intake with cans of cola and their dairy intake with ice cream, you can say with confidence that a significant increase in inflammatory markers would be present after just a couple of weeks.

The bottom line: Although increasing added or refined sugar intake does not independently cause inflammation in a controlled setting, it *can* contribute to an increase in systemic inflammation when that consumption is accompanied by other pro-inflammatory habits, or when that increase in sugar intake leads to increased adiposity (body fat), visceral adiposity and weight gain. Focusing on consuming sugars found in more nutrient-rich foods, such as fruit and dairy, is always a good idea.

Inflammation myth no. 4: Gluten is best avoided

Contemplating going gluten-free? Well, you wouldn't be the first. In the UK alone, it's estimated that 8 million people follow a gluten-free diet, with the majority of them classified as PWAGs (people without coeliac disease avoiding gluten). This is in part attributed to a dramatic proliferation of social media posts and advertisements stating that gluten is inflammatory or damaging to the gut. So, does going gluten-free really benefit your health, or is it just a widely amplified fad?

Gluten is a group of proteins found in many grains, such as wheat and barley. Typical foods containing gluten include bread, pasta and various cereals. Coeliac disease is a common condition that affects roughly 1 per cent of the population.[19] This is an auto-immune condition in which the small intestine is hypersensitive to gluten. In people with coeliac disease, it is of course essential to avoid gluten to ameliorate symptoms and inflammation, and improve gut health and life expectancy.

There is also a group of people who experience negative symptoms when eating gluten, but who have normal blood-test and biopsy results. These people are classified as having non-coeliac gluten sensitivity (NCGS), which has a prevalence only marginally greater than coeliac disease.[20] Common symptoms include abdominal pain, bloating, diarrhoea, constipation, various aches, fatigue and joint pain. Sometimes it can be caused by a wheat allergy, linked to irritable bowel syndrome (IBS), but typically medical experts are not sure why it occurs. There is also a subset of people with other autoimmune conditions such as Hashi-moto's thyroiditis, who may see an improvement in blood test results and symptoms by avoiding gluten.[21] This is because the antibodies that attack the thyroid in someone with Hashimoto's do not distinguish between the protein structures of gluten and the thyroid. However, the research is mixed, and as we'll soon see, a gluten-free diet may actually increase inflammatory potential, so this is a highly individualized conversation that should be reserved for you and your doctor. Generally, if certain foods cause you negative symptoms, it is probably wise to avoid them, regardless of a diagnosis.

You might be wondering: *If I'm not coeliac or experiencing nega-tive symptoms, is gluten-free really better for me?* To answer this, let me first clarify that there is limited objective clinical evidence demonstrating that gluten causes inflammation in those without coeliac disease. Interestingly, though, some data shows that avoiding gluten without a medical need can have *adverse* health effects, such as increased blood pressure and an increased risk of coronary artery disease.[22] A large trial comprising the Nurses' Health Study and the Health Professionals Follow-up Study cohorts followed 100,000 people for twenty-six years.[23] Researchers found that long-term consumption of gluten was not associated with coronary heart disease, while avoiding it resulted in reduced whole-grain consumption, which may in fact increase your risk of disease. The teams concluded that following a gluten-free diet without coeliac disease was not advisable. Further to this, people following gluten-free diets are typically at an increased risk of nutrient deficiencies, including in fibre, iron, calcium and magnesium.[24]

Some people, even some carnivorously inclined medical doctors, argue that gluten causes gut inflammation, in that it supposedly facilitates dysfunction in the tight junctions that play an important role in intestinal barrier function.[25] This has been said to cause an unsubstantiated, pseudoscientific condition called 'leaky gut'. In a recent study of 160,000 US women, which assessed the risk of microscopic colitis (inflammation of the lower GI tract) with consumption of gluten,[26] once again researchers found no link between inflammatory processes in the gut and gluten in the diet. We will learn about the importance of the Dietary Inflammatory Index (DII) in determining a diet's capacity to induce systemic inflammation, and how this recent study highlights an interesting point. As part of the study, twenty-three healthy women were put on a gluten-free diet for six weeks.[27] Compared to the women's usual diet, the gluten-free diet increased the DII score – increasing the diet's inflammatory potential, due to the absence of key nutrients from whole grains (like polyphenols, minerals and fibre).

The bottom line: There is limited evidence that the consumption of gluten causes inflammation, either systemically or locally within the gut. In fact, the evidence points to the contrary – avoiding gluten without a medical need to do so can increase your risk of cardiovascular disease, weight gain, nutrient deficiencies and inflammation. Not to mention that it can hurt your bank account too! Gluten-free foods are on average 242 per cent more expensive than their regular counterparts.[28] So, unless you have coeliac disease, gluten sensitivity or an allergy – or another autoimmune condition whereby avoiding gluten is a medical recommendation – you may be causing yourself more harm than good by avoiding gluten.

Inflammation myth no. 5: Weight gain and inflammation aren't connected

Various factors can contribute to chronic inflammation, including age, diet, whether a person is a smoker, stress, insufficient sleep and hormonal imbalances.[29] However, excess adiposity, or weight gain, is strongly associated with chronic inflammation and is thought to be one of the main reasons that obesity entails health risks.[30]

When energy intake exceeds energy output, the size and number of fat cells will grow, and body fat levels will start to accumulate. As they continue to grow, the cells may eventually rupture, resulting in an inflammatory response.[31] Evidence suggests several other intricate factors are at play here. One study took gluteal fat biopsies from both obese and normal-weighted individuals.[32] Researchers examined the small arteries within these samples of tissue, and found that the tissue from the normal-weighted subjects secreted chemical messengers that induced vasodilation (expansion) of the vessels to help nutrients reach cells, whereas the fat from obese subjects had a loss of this dilator effect, accompanied by an increase of TNF-a receptors (TNF-a being an inflammatory cytokine). The implication of this is an inability to supply cells with adequate levels of oxygen, which is thought to be a major driver of adipose tissue dysfunction – known as local hypoxia, or the 'starving' of oxygen. This process leads to cell death, oxidative stress, cellular rupture and a reduction in anti-inflammatory hormones such as adiponectin, all of which contribute to chronic inflammation.

The association between weight gain and inflammation is of course closely tied to what and how much a person eats. A diet that is lacking in nutrient-dense foods and is rich in certain types of ultra-processed foods makes gaining weight infinitely easier. It just so happens that many foods that contribute to weight gain are also high on the DII, and so are characterized as pro-inflammatory.[33] This compounds the effect that these foods have on chronic inflammation in the body. It is extremely easy to consume refined sugars in excess; foods that are 'hyper-palatable' (ultra-processed, high-fat, high-sugar, high-salt, or a combination of the three) trigger certain reward centres in the brain, making going back for a second portion a simple decision. Conversely, natural sugars aren't really the issue; when's the last time you observed someone becoming obese from eating lots of fruit?

The bottom line: Weight gain is an important player in chronic inflammation for several reasons. Excess fat tissue releases pro-inflammatory chemicals, influences hormone release and is closely tied to poorer food choices, all of which impact inflammation. Managing your weight will have a crucial anti-inflammatory benefit, irrespective of your food choices.

A deeper dive

Having dispelled some prevalent myths about diet and inflammation so far in this chapter, it's essential to ground our understanding in the solid foundation of scientific evidence. So let's delve into the intricacies of inflammation at a cellular level, and explore the dietary patterns proven to mitigate its harmful effects.

Back in AD 25, the Roman scholar Celsus defined the four classical signs of inflammation: *rubor*, *dolor*, *calor* and *tumor* (meaning 'redness', 'pain', 'heat' and 'swelling').[34] These four words characterize inflammation's earliest clinical symptoms. Put simply, they are what you experience after you roll over on your ankle. Inflammation is an essential part of healing and life, and is present even in single-cell organisms like bacteria.

Chronic versus acute inflammation

When the internal inflammatory battle wages on for more than a few days, however, irreversible and long-lasting damage can be done to your body. This is called chronic inflammation, and is when things become a problem. When inflammation becomes chronic – or for more accurate phrasing, when it becomes 'chronic low-grade systemic inflammation' (meaning throughout the whole body) – there's hell to pay. I'm looking at you, cardiovascular disease, inflammatory bowel disease (IBD), arthritis and even dementia.

As the name implies, chronic inflammation is long-lasting. Unfortunately, it is neither easily resolved nor quickly reversed. Chronic inflammation begins insidiously and may result from exposure to a low-intensity irritant, toxin or microbe, or it can be the consequence of autoimmunity, as seen in conditions such as IBD. However, it's becoming increasingly clear that the specific constituents of our diet have a profound effect on not just chronic, systemic inflammation, but also our ability to mount an acute inflammatory response.

Altering the ratio of certain nutrients can aid in the anti-inflammatory potential of our diet. For example, replacing saturated fatty acids with omega-3 fatty acids, or adding spices and herbs like garlic and pepper to our meals, can tremendously reduce inflammation (topics we will dive into later). It's crucial to highlight that while the large majority of the scientific discussion concerns diet and *chronic* inflammation, we will briefly touch on how to optimize the *acute* inflammatory response to help us overcome illness and trauma in the short term.

Inflammation and cardiovascular disease

Cardiovascular disease, which includes diseases of the heart and vessels, is the world's single biggest killer. We've known for several decades that inflammation damages the lining of the vessels and heart tissue and plays a vital role in the build-up of plaque within arteries (on top of cholesterol). The irony is that the chronic inflammation that damages the arteries then leads to more inflammation at the site of injury, and a vicious cycle ensues.

Among the scientific community, no one was really sure whether inflammation could only load, or also light, the cannon on heart attacks or strokes – until a few years ago. A large randomized controlled trial studied over 10,000 patients who had previously suffered heart attacks and had high levels of inflammation (CRP > 2mg/L).[35] The researchers were testing whether the drug canakinumab, an anti-inflammatory medication that targets the inflammatory cytokine interleukin-1β, was able to reduce the risk of a repeat cardiovascular 'event'. Patients receiving the drug were found to have a greatly reduced rate of recurrent heart attack or stroke. This was a sweet vindication for the cardiovascular research team, who had long suspected that inflammation was as important as cholesterol in heart disease.

The Dietary Inflammatory Index (DII)

A professor at the University of South Carolina, Dr James Hébert, once described how, growing up, he would always get injured while playing sport. Little hamstring niggles, joint issues, muscle strains and the like. He then made the peculiar observation that his injuries would heal much faster towards the end of summer compared to the winter and autumn months. Why was this happening?

As a child, Hébert used to help his parents grow and plant certain crops in the garden, such as beans, vegetables and fruit. These crops would only come into season during the summer months, and during that time he would feast on these rich and diverse plant foods. It was only several decades later that he realized what was happening: the nutrients in these foods were aiding the healing process during the summer months. In 2009, Dr Hébert created what we know today as the Dietary Inflammatory Index (DII). Simply put, if you understand the DII, you understand how diet affects inflammation in the body.

The DII is an innovative scoring system that uses the inflammatory properties of dietary components to estimate the overall inflammatory potential of an individual's diet.[36] What Hébert and his team did was go and identify databases around the world that included surveys from different countries with vastly different dietary habits. They merged heaps of data and formed a composite data set that gave individual nutrients a value ranging from –1 (being the most anti-inflammatory) to 1 (most inflammatory possible), with a score of 0 meaning no effect on bodily inflammation at all.

Which foods reign king?

There are many diets that can be considered 'anti-inflammatory', and virtually all of them focus on plant-based eating. To illustrate this, here are the DII scores of some popular dietary patterns today, which combine the nutrient values of each diet and give a combined DII score (remember, negative numbers = anti-inflammatory):[37]

1. The Mediterranean diet = –2.92
2. Mayo clinic = –3.22
3. Paleo diet = –3.42
4. Vegan diet = –3.87
5. Ornish diet = –4.52
6. Biggest Loser = –4.52

The dietary patterns that are the most anti-inflammatory tend to have the highest concentration of foods that are highly pigmented and flavourful. These foods are calorie-sparse and nutrient-dense. This is crucial to the mediating effect that body habitus (meaning the physical characteristics of a body) has on inflammation.

Simply put, because overconsuming food and gaining weight is inflammatory by nature, it makes sense that calorie-sparse foods can help to reduce inflammation. It's possible to increase the anti-inflammatory capacity of the diet by replacing calorie-dense, refined, pro-inflammatory foods that tend to lack natural flavour, colour and aroma with highly pigmented and flavourful ones. Below is a breakdown of the key nutrients and compounds that have anti-inflammatory potential.

Anti-inflammatory compounds present in food tend to fit within these groups:

- **Plant foods** – In particular herbs and spices, like pepper, garlic, onion, rosemary, thyme, ginger and black and green tea.
- **Classes of polyphenols** – Isoflavones, flavonoids and anthocyanidins are found in large quantities within berries, dark leafy greens and cruciferous vegetables.
- **Vitamins, minerals and antioxidants** – These are found concentrated in fruits and vegetables.
- **Unsaturated fatty acids** – Omega-3 fats have the most powerful anti-inflammatory effect relative to dose and are found in sea or land plants, and in the animals that eat them (like fatty fish).

Although we don't have room to explain how every single food group or compound is anti- or pro-inflammatory, here are the mechanisms behind a few of them to give you an initial understanding.

FLAVONOIDS (ANTI-INFLAMMATORY)

Flavonoids belong to the group of compounds called polyphenols, which have a wide range of biological benefits – including antioxidant, anti-inflammatory, antiviral and anti-mutagenic properties.[38] The highest dietary sources of flavonoids include berries, leafy vegetables, onions, soybeans, tea and dark chocolate.

One recent study showed that consuming just 123g of a raspberry smoothie every day for two weeks significantly reduced CRP in patients with type 2 diabetes.[39] This happened because of the ability of the flavonoids' hydroxyl groups (one oxygen bonded to one hydrogen atom) to scavenge and stabilize free radicals and reduce oxidative damage, both of which are key to initiating the negative effects of chronic inflammation.[40]

Because flavonoids possess anti-inflammatory properties, they also serve as potent anti-cancer phytochemicals. They work through several mechanisms, such as triggering cell-cycle arrest, the induction of apoptosis (cellular death) in cancer cells[41] and the inhibition of angiogenesis (the formation of new blood vessels, which is crucial in cancer growth). Flavonoids have been shown to inhibit tumour-cell proliferation via the inhibition of enzymes like COX-2, xanthine oxidase and 5-LOX, which are major catalysts responsible for tumour progression.

BETA-CAROTENE (ANTI-INFLAMMATORY)

Dietary carotenoids (of which beta-carotene is the most well known) are found in many yellow, orange and green leafy fruits and vegetables such as carrots, corn, red bell peppers and mangoes. Carotenoids are the most abundant lipid-soluble phytochemicals, and research has shown them to have strong anti-inflammatory properties. This has been attributed to their ability to block the translocation (a type of genetic change) of nuclear factor kB (NF-kB) to the cell nucleus. This disrupts the NF-kB pathway, thus inhibiting the production of inflammatory cytokines such as interleukin-8 and prostaglandin E2.[42]

SATURATED FATS (PRO-INFLAMMATORY)

Several studies have demonstrated that saturated fats – found in high quantities in foods like butter, cakes and processed meats – initiate inflammation in fat tissue. This happens because of the stimulation of Toll-like Receptor 4 (TLR4),[43] which plays a key role in the innate immune response. Toll-like receptors also increase the expression of inflammatory genes. Saturated fatty acids also enhance the activation of transcription factors (proteins that alter gene expression) such as NF-kB, which is involved in inflammatory and immune responses, as well as the regulation of other genes related to cell survival and proliferation. A study on overweight men found that consuming 50g of butter leads to significant increases in interleukin-6, which is an inflammatory cytokine.[44]

Diet and acute inflammation

While we've talked a lot about how to suppress chronic inflammation, the ability to mount an inflammatory response in order to recover from an injury is also worth a brief discussion. There are two distinct phases in the body's response to an injury: the initiation and the resolution of inflammation. This process has been termed the 'Resolution Response' by Dr Barry Sears.[45] The key dietary principles that optimize the Resolution Response – and therefore acute inflammation – include a dietary pattern that is calorie-restricted, low in fat, sufficient in protein and rich in omega-3 fatty acids and polyphenols. These are some of the key dietary components to consider in order to optimize your ability to recover from an injury.

Calorie restriction

The most important consideration for any anti-inflammatory diet is caloric restriction, which in essence means avoiding overeating. This will lead to a significant decrease in systemic oxidative stress. Calorie restriction has been the most successful therapeutic intervention to improve health span (defined as the number of years someone lives without disability or illness) in virtually every animal and human model studied.[46] A perfect example of this is the two-year CALERIE study,[47] which showed that a twenty-five per cent reduction in calories leads to improved cardiometabolic blood markers, as well as a significant reduction in CRP. This is why simply reducing the amount of food you eat is a potent anti-inflammatory strategy which helps the body to quickly recover from an acute injury. Eating too much food, or gaining excess adipose tissue, causes excess circulating free fatty acids in the bloodstream, and these turn on pro-inflammatory signals. This is one of the reasons that obesity is so strongly associated with inflammation and is linked to many chronic inflammatory disease states.

Protein

Dietary protein plays an important role in the acute inflammatory response, by providing the body with the necessary building blocks to synthesize and maintain the immune system's components.[48] During inflammation, the body's immune system is activated, which leads to an increased demand for protein. Proteins are required to produce cytokines, which tell the immune system to respond to inflammation. Protein is also needed to produce antibodies, which target and neutralize harmful pathogens –

as well as white blood cells, which are important components of the immune system. Inflammation can lead to tissue damage, therefore protein is similarly needed for the synthesis of new tissue and the repair of damaged tissue. This is especially important in cases of acute injury, where protein can help speed up the healing process and minimize the risk of infection.[49] Overall, dietary protein is essential for supporting the immune system and aiding in the body's response to inflammation. It is important to consume adequate amounts of protein to ensure proper immune function and tissue repair.[50]

Omega-3 fatty acids

Omega-3 fatty acids have been shown to reduce levels of inflammation through various mechanisms. One of the most well-known is the inhibition of the production of pro-inflammatory cytokines and chemokines, which activate the immune system and contribute to inflammation.[51] Studies have found that omega-3s can reduce the production of cytokines such as interleukin-6 (IL-6) and interleukin-1 (IL-1).[52] They can also inhibit the activation of certain transcription factors that enhance inflammation and they reduce the production of reactive oxygen species, which further lessens inflammation.[53] These mechanisms contribute to the overall anti-inflammatory effects of omega-3 fatty acids and help to explain their potential benefits in reducing inflammation and its associated health problems.

Polyphenols

We now know that many micronutrients and polyphenolic compounds (such as flavonoids) are not just strongly anti-inflammatory in the long term, but also promote competent pro-inflammatory signalling with respect to acute inflammation. These nutrients alter the actions of NF-kB, AMP-activated protein kinase (AMPK), eicosanoids and resolvins, which are all key mediators of inflammatory processes.[54]

Key takeaways

1. **Avoid overconsuming food!** The single best dietary thing you can do to reduce inflammation is to restrict your calorie intake. This means focusing on foods that are going to satiate and satisfy you in order to prevent overeating and weight gain. Calorie restriction has been demonstrated to be strongly anti-inflammatory in every randomized controlled trial conducted on humans. This is why simply reducing the amount of food you eat, irrespective of whether you change *what* you're eating, is a potent anti-inflammatory strategy.

2. **Taste the rainbow!** Foods that are colourful, full of taste and nutrient-dense are key. This is because these foods contain many compounds that are strongly anti-inflammatory. Some key foods to consider include:

   - *A berry good idea!* Eat a small bowl of berries (such as blueberries, blackberries and raspberries) regularly. These are rich in flavonoids and various antioxidants, which are strongly anti-inflammatory and essential in the repair and resolution of the inflammatory response. Eating 250g of blueberries a day has been shown to reduce oxidative stress and increase anti-inflammatory cytokines in well-trained athletes.[55]
   - *Finish your veg!* Kale, parsley, red cabbage, onions and dark leafy greens are extremely rich in flavonoids and various vitamins and minerals, which are also anti-inflammatory.

- *Add some spice!* Herbs and spices can always be added to food, teas, salads etc., not just for flavour but for their incredible anti-inflammatory effect. Turmeric, ginger, cayenne pepper, chillies and even green tea are potently anti-inflammatory and will suppress bodily inflammation.

3. **Go easy on the fried stuff!** Fried foods are typically high in saturated and trans-unsaturated fatty acids, which have consistently been shown to be pro-inflammatory. But remember, the dose is what matters. One serving of fried food a week will likely not affect systemic inflammation in the context of your overall dietary pattern.

4. **Sugar-free all day!** If you're the type to enjoy a nice can of sugary pop, or a slice of cake in the evenings, one of the most healthful habits you can engage in is to reduce your consumption of added sugars, especially in combination with these other changes. This will help you manage your total calorie intake. Look to sugars found in fruits and dairy to fulfil your sweet cravings and ease your inflammatory worries.

5. **Bulk up the omega-3s!** Foods high in omega-3s such as fatty fish, olive oil, flaxseed, chia seeds and walnuts play a vital role in reducing inflammasome activity, which stimulates the release of pro-inflammatory cytokines such as interleukins.

Weight

The Big Fat Debate

The effect that diet has on bodily inflammation is a critical and much misunderstood topic, but I now want to turn to an even more controversial area of health and nutrition: the subject of fat. At any given time, 45 per cent of people are actively trying to lose weight.[1] Unsurprisingly, as we'll see, most of those attempts end up in failure. In this chapter, I'll break down what it means to be overweight and the consequences on your body of carrying excess fat. I'll debunk some common myths surrounding weight loss and shed light on how to get rid of the most harmful type of fat in the body: visceral fat. This subject will also be explored further in the weight-loss chapter, where I'll provide a critical overview of my best evidence-based strategies to lose body fat and keep it off for good.

What do you think of when you hear the word 'fat'? Stripping the concept of fat to its rawest form, what we're really referring to are individual cells called adipocytes, which when found together are known as adipose tissue. These cells are fundamental to the survival of all mammals – from bears to camels to humans.

Adipocytes have three main functions. First, they act as an energy bank. In times of low energy, adipocytes can be broken down into triglycerides and release free fatty acids (FFAs), which can then be burned for energy. Second, a type of adipocyte present in mammals serves to produce heat. These 'brown adipocytes' have thermogenic properties due to mitochondria within the cell; the mitochondria are also responsible for its colour. Historically, these brown cells protect mammals against the cold and are often referred to as the 'hibernating organ', but they also function in response to exercise and in pathological conditions (disease or abnormal bodily state) to help regulate body temperature. Third, adipocytes produce hormones to influence energy intake. Leptin, for example, is a central hormone that regulates satiety and is produced and secreted by adipocytes.

Another hormone, adiponectin, also released from adipocytes, plays a critical role in protecting against insulin resistance and atherosclerosis.[2] While adipocytes are essential to life, carrying excessive amounts of adipose tissue causes health issues – and this is what is implied when someone is colloquially labelled 'fat'. Globally, around 13 per cent of people are classified as obese, rising to 25 per cent in countries such as the UK. And in the USA, despite having the highest worldwide expenditure on healthcare, a whopping 43 per cent of US adults and 20 per cent of children are obese.[3]

It's logical to conclude that the physical burden of lugging too much weight around comes with inherent risk. Did you know that every pound of excess fat exerts a four-fold burden on your knee per step during daily activities?[4] And too much fat around the neck can compress the trachea and suffocate you in your sleep, known as obstructive sleep apnoea. Individuals with obesity also struggle with issues related to their mood, self-esteem, quality of life and body image.[5] Many of my patients who are overweight have described the discomfort and pain they experience with every thigh-chafing step, which may not seem like a big deal to some but can be debilitating for those living with it every day.

Clearly the physical burden of excess body fat is a problem, but it's not the only downside. The biochemical products of fat tissue are where things get sticky, literally. Think of fat as an endocrine organ – that is, any organ that produces and secretes hormones. Just like the pituitary, thyroid or adrenal gland, fat tissue is much the same in that it regulates certain hormonal functions. In the last chapter, we saw how when we have too much fat tissue, it can cause local hypoxia, reduced blood flow and adipocyte cell death – which releases harmful pro-inflammatory and pro-thrombotic (clot-forming) chemicals into the bloodstream. These processes greatly increase your risk of cardiovascular and metabolic diseases and various types of cancer, as well as mental health disorders like depression. But is obesity actually harmful? Isn't it all just association and not causation? Isn't attempting weight loss futile because the majority of diets fail? Doesn't weight loss bring out more harm than good? Isn't BMI racist?

Before we tackle these questions and dive into the science of obesity and how to combat it, it's important to establish whether obesity even poses a risk to our health.

Weight myth no. 1: It's possible to be obese and not be at risk of disease in later life

Obesity is typically defined as an abnormal or excessive accumulation of fat that presents a health risk, with a BMI >30. The health risks of obesity are arguably one of the most well-established fields of health science in the literature. Obesity contributes to a reduced life expectancy and impaired quality of life, due to an increased risk of many diseases including cardiovascular disease,[6] type 2 diabetes,[7] osteoarthritis,[8] mental health disorders[9] and cancer.*[10]

Most importantly, these increases in disease risk aren't small, either. They surpass the magnitude of effect from any dietary

---

* These aren't just links by association, but also Mendelian randomization (MR), which analyses genetic variation to infer causation. Just to highlight how extensive the evidence base is, the citation I have included for cardiovascular disease alone examined 53 meta-analyses and over 500 individual research studies, along with several MR genetic analyses. The citation for diabetes analysed over 216 studies, including 2.3 million people.

habit you can think of. Some meta-analyses show that people with a BMI of more than 30 have a 628 per cent increased risk of type 2 diabetes even after adjusting for age, family history and physical activity.[11] That far and away surpasses the risks that come from being inactive, sleeping poorly, eating fried foods and even alcohol consumption. Obesity is the second leading cause of cancer in the UK after smoking, increasing the risk of thirteen types of cancer including liver, kidney, thyroid, ovarian and breast cancer by up to 100 per cent.[12] In comparison, having a diet high in carbohydrates and fatty foods would increase your risk of certain cancers by just 35 per cent.[13]

If you are obese, it's entirely possible to improve your health by moving more, engaging in exercise, managing sleep and stress and making better dietary choices without ever losing weight. These habits can even normalize your metabolic blood tests, known as metabolically healthy obesity (MHO). Healthy blood results in these cases would indicate good health at that time, for several different reasons. For one, people engaging in these healthful behaviours may have a lower proportion of visceral fat, preserved insulin sensitivity and beta-cell function, and improved cardiorespiratory fitness compared to unhealthy obese individuals.[14] Incorporating health-promoting habits should absolutely be the priority.

Nevertheless, even if all of your blood tests are normal yet you remain obese, unfortunately you will still have an increased risk of chronic diseases in the long run. One study looked at 3.5 million people and followed them over five years. Compared to normal-weighted individuals, MHO people still had a 49 per cent increased risk of coronary heart disease and a higher risk of heart failure.[15] The same is seen in dozens of other studies, which conclude that the term 'metabolically healthy obesity' should be avoided as it is misleading.[16] This is why incorporating health-promoting behaviours *and* aiming for sustainable weight loss are key pillars to longevity and health. Remember that even if you don't achieve long-term weight loss, *any* period of time at a lower weight is still beneficial, demonstrated in an analysis of 161,000 people concluding that every additional weight-loss attempt of >5lbs further reduces your risk of death even if you regain the weight.[17]

The bottom line: Obesity increases your risk of many diseases and cancers by an alarming amount. It's encouraged to engage in healthy lifestyle habits regardless of your weight, however even if you do exercise, eat well and have normal blood tests, being obese still puts you at an increased risk of disease in later life.

Weight myth no. 2: BMI is racist

The criticism that Body Mass Index (BMI) is useless and even racist stems from concerns about the universal application of a measurement system that doesn't consider the diverse body compositions, ethnic backgrounds and health risks among different populations. The roots of BMI trace back to the nineteenth century, when it was created by the Belgian mathematician Lambert Adolphe Jacques Quetelet. It was initially designed to measure populations, not individuals, and was further developed by Ancel Keys in the 1960s and 1970s.

Its formula (weight in kilograms divided by height in metres squared) was based on predominantly white European populations, and therefore critics argue that it doesn't necessarily apply to all ethnic and racial groups. Research shows that different ethnic groups have varying risks of health conditions at the same BMI.[18] For instance, people of Asian descent tend to have higher body-fat percentages and risk of conditions like heart disease and diabetes at lower BMIs than people of European descent. Conversely, people of African descent may have lower risks of these conditions at the same or higher BMIs than their white counterparts.

So it is true that when it comes to health, a high BMI doesn't necessarily tell you the full story. The more accurate classification of obesity is >25 per cent body fat for men and >30 per cent for women. Despite these limitations, the validation studies prove that BMI is very closely correlated with increasing body-fat percentage across populations from all over the world.[19] Interestingly, in a Sri Lankan cohort, for example, everyone (both men and women) who had a BMI above 30 also had a body-fat percentage that would define obesity (>25 per cent for men and >30 per cent for women), so clearly the measurement's ability to predict body-fat percentage is strong.[20] The fact is, we still see increasing disease risk in the obese cohort across the world. Therefore, the way you label BMI is irrelevant as it still highlights an at-risk population that would benefit from lifestyle intervention.

The bottom line: The important thing to remember is that BMI shouldn't be used in isolation to predict someone's health risk. This is really the case with any objective health measurement (whether it's blood pressure, fasting glucose, heart rate, estimated glomerular filtration rate to check for kidney function or full blood count), as they're all pretty useless by themselves. In isolation they tell you very little, yet when these measurements are assessed together with BMI, they can and do inform the diagnostic work-up and clinical course for an individual – allowing for an accurate depiction of future health risk.

Weight myth no. 3: Weight loss does more harm than good

Often, people who make this claim cite studies apparently showing that losing weight increases the risk of death from cardiovascular disease, diabetes or even mental health disorders.[21] This is a fundamental error in research interpretation, as the key issue here is whether the weight loss is intentional or not.

Unintentional weight loss is one of the most dangerous

symptoms we look out for as doctors, as it's usually suggestive of an underlying malignancy, serious metabolic or autoimmune disease or an illness that's so debilitating it completely halts appetite or prevents eating. In this context, losing weight is often an indicator of someone nearing death, so it's not surprising that *unintentional* weight loss would be associated with an increase in mortality risk.

The bottom line: Of course, some people experience negative effects from intentional weight loss if they follow a method lacking in balance, flexibility and scientific backing. However, for most people with obesity, dozens of controlled trials show that intentional weight loss is consistently linked to improved physical and mental health outcomes.[22]

Weight myth no. 4: The benefits of weight loss are solely down to changing lifestyle habits, not the weight loss itself

The Health at Every Size (HAES) movement emerged as a response to traditional approaches to health that focused largely on body weight. Advocates argue for a holistic understanding of health that goes beyond just the number on the scale. They contend that overall wellness can be enhanced through lifestyle changes, regardless of whether weight loss occurs. According to HAES supporters, weight loss may simply be a side effect of adopting healthier habits, not the primary driver of improved health.

This viewpoint, however, doesn't fully capture the complexity of health outcomes related to weight. To illustrate this, let's consider a controlled study that specifically tested the connection between dietary habits, weight loss and health.[23] Two groups of women were given diets that were identical in calories, protein, carbs and fats, ensuring that both would lose weight. The key difference was their sugar intake – one group consumed 120g of table sugar each day, while the other had only 11g. Despite the high sugar consumption, which most health professionals would advise against, both groups experienced weight loss, lowered blood pressure and improved blood lipids.

This experiment demonstrates that even when a lifestyle change doesn't necessarily promote health – in this case, consuming a high-sugar diet – the associated weight loss can still have beneficial effects on various health markers.

The bottom line: The relationship between lifestyle changes, weight loss and health is more nuanced than the HAES perspective might imply. While the movement rightly emphasizes the importance of lifestyle modifications for overall health, it's also crucial to acknowledge that weight loss itself can contribute to better health outcomes, even when it's achieved through less-than-optimal lifestyle changes. Therefore, a comprehensive approach to health should consider both lifestyle habits and weight management.

Weight myth no. 5: Pursuing weight loss is futile

The idea that 'as 95 per cent of diets fail' it's not worth trying to lose weight is one of the most prevalent and damaging misconceptions perpetuated by the anti-diet or HAES community. It's extremely disheartening to see even a large number of medical doctors and registered dietitians perpetuating this statistic on social media.

Let's clear something up first. The '95 per cent' statistic came from a single study undertaken back in 1959, when 100 people were given a random 'diet' to follow and then sent on their way. With no ongoing support or guidance, I'd expect them to fail! Many decades later, ironically even the author of that study told the *New York Times* that the study had little relevance and 'I've been sort of surprised that people keep citing it.'[24]

When it comes to characterizing a diet as having 'failed' or 'succeeded', we need to be realistic in our goals and redefine what it means to 'succeed' at weight loss. If you're a 40-year-old mum with two kids and a full-time job, it's probably not realistic to define success as getting back to your 23-year-old, responsibility-free, six-gym-sessions-a-week, chiselled frame. Life changes. Priorities change. People have families and responsibilities, and may be working so much they barely have time to sleep.

You need to go easy on yourself, be understanding and practise some self-compassion. Did you know that it only takes 5–10 per cent weight loss in those who are overweight to see clinically meaningful improvements in health? At just 2.5 per cent weight loss we begin to see improvements in menstrual irregularities and fertility, which is especially important in polycystic ovarian syndrome. At 5 per cent weight loss we see improvements in glycaemic control, which is especially important for those who are insulin-resistant or type 2 diabetic. When you hit 5–10 per cent weight loss, we see meaningful improvements in blood pressure and blood lipids, both of which are crucial to cardiovascular health. Then, at around 15 per cent weight loss, we start to notice substantial improvements in sleep apnoea and non-alcoholic fatty liver disease.[25]

Seeing that the definition of obesity is 'excess weight that poses a risk to health', these improvements in health outcomes should be the real definition of weight-loss success. These thresholds are realistic and *have* been demonstrated in meta-analyses of twenty-nine randomized controlled trials,[26] showing that those who initially lose >20kg (44lbs) managed to maintain over 7kg (15lbs) of weight loss after five years.* So, losing weight long-term

---

* Perhaps most notably the Look AHEAD (Action for Health in Diabetes) trial in 2014, which was a multi-centre RCT done at sixteen clinical sites in the USA. They recruited 5,145 obese adults with type 2 diabetes and assigned patients to an intensive lifestyle intervention that included regular behavioural weight-loss counselling. They saw that >50 per cent of those with support along the journey maintained >5 per cent weight loss and 25 per cent maintained >10 per cent weight loss after eight years. These statistics were even larger in those who lost >10 per cent of body weight in the first year (65 and 39 per cent respectively).

can be seriously beneficial for your health and *is* achievable, even if it's just a little at first.

The one important caveat I would highlight is that during any weight-loss programme, you should ensure adequate levels of protein intake (>1.6g/kg), and resistance training should be encouraged to minimize the loss of lean mass.

The bottom line: Based on lots of previous trials, losing a meaningful amount of weight over a prolonged period with the purpose of improving health outcomes is very achievable and should be encouraged for all people with obesity.

Weight myth no. 6: All body fat is equal

This may come as a surprise to many of you, but excess body fat isn't really the issue when it comes to obesity; the issue is excess *visceral* fat. What do we mean by this? Visceral fat (or intra-abdominal adipose tissue) is a specific type of fat that sits deep inside the abdomen, with unique metabolic properties. It also pushes our belly outwards, in contrast to subcutaneous fat that lies just beneath the skin and which you see and feel everywhere on your body.

So what's the issue with visceral fat? It functions like an endocrine organ and draws considerable interest from endocrinologists. Its ability to produce hormones, interfere with insulin signalling, release pro-inflammatory cytokines and disrupt organ functionality has caused concern. Furthermore, the prevalence of glucocorticoid and androgen receptors (two types of hormonal receptors), as well as inflammatory and immune cells, makes visceral fat more insulin-resistant, sensitive to lipolysis (breakdown of fat), metabolically active and prone to releasing free fatty acids.[27] This explains why each additional 'excess' inch on your waist independently increases your risk of death by 2.75 per cent, even if you appear slim elsewhere.[28] The focus of our discussion will now shift to the key strategies that can specifically target and reduce this harmful visceral fat, even without overall weight loss.

Engaging in cardiovascular exercises like running, cycling, rowing and swimming is uniquely effective in dissipating visceral fat. These activities result in a prolonged period of effort and a high heart rate. Over 100 randomized controlled trials comparing dieting with exercise found that only exercise led to a 6 per cent reduction in visceral fat without weight loss.[29] You might be wondering, surely strength training does the same thing, though? I'm sorry to tell you that it doesn't.[30] This is due to strength training largely revolving around long rest periods, shorter periods of intensity and typically less calorie-burn.

So how does cardio target visceral fat? Cardio stimulates interleukin-6, which aids in visceral fat breakdown,* and due to visceral fat's metabolic activity it's more sensitive to sympathetic activation (fight-or-flight response), making cardio more effective in stimulating its lipolysis.[31] Interestingly, studies often show a reduction in visceral fat while total body fat stays the same, indicating that cardio 'burns' visceral fat and redistributes it to less harmful subcutaneous areas. This fact is evident in sumo wrestlers, who despite their high-calorie intake and obesity, maintain healthy glucose, triglyceride, and metabolic blood levels because their extensive cardiovascular exercise redistributes visceral fat.[32]

Doing 3–4 weekly sessions of moderate- to high-intensity cardio lasting 30–60 minutes each has been shown to be effective

---

* Interleukin-6 is a complex cytokine that plays a role in both pro-inflammatory and anti-inflammatory pathways. In acute inflammatory situations, such as infection or injury, IL-6 is produced by various cells (like macrophages) and acts to initiate an inflammatory response. But IL-6 also has a role in regulating inflammatory responses. It participates in the induction of a class of T-cells called regulatory T-cells that suppress immune responses, preventing excessive inflammation and autoimmunity.

for visceral fat loss.[33] A simple way to figure out what constitutes a 'moderate' intensity exercise is to first find your maximum heart rate (220 minus your age), then to find 65–75 per cent of that. For example, if you're forty years old, 0.65 x 180 = 117, therefore your cardio should be stimulating a heart rate of >117 to be considered 'moderate' intensity.

Various other factors can influence the storage of visceral fat in the body. Consuming foods with high glycaemic loads (e.g. those rich in refined sugars and lacking in fibre or fats, like sweets and sugary drinks) or foods which are high in saturated fats has been shown to increase visceral fat. Reducing total glycaemic load can result in an 11 per cent reduction in abdominal fat without weight loss,[34] while saturated fats tend to store intrahepatic triglycerides (IHTGs) and increase liver fat. This, in turn, spills over into the rest of the abdominal cavity, increasing visceral fat stores. One study showed that when people are overfed 1,000kcal/day of different nutrients for three weeks, the saturated fat group increased IHTGs by 55 per cent, the simple sugars group increased IHTGs by 33 per cent, and the unsaturated fat group 15 per cent.[35] Alcohol consumption is also closely linked to visceral fat levels, as alcohol damages the liver, affects nutrient metabolism and storage, and reduces testosterone levels.[36] Stress and cortisol are similarly linked, and cortisol has been shown to redistribute fat stores towards the abdomen, increase appetite and reduce post-meal energy expenditure.[37]

The bottom line: Visceral fat is worse for overall health than subcutaneous fat. To reduce visceral fat, it is advisable to engage in regular moderate- or high-intensity cardiovascular exercise, and to replace high-glycaemic-load and saturated fatty foods with fibrous carbohydrates (e.g. fruits, vegetables and whole grains) and unsaturated fats. Similarly, limiting alcohol consumption and engaging in stress-relieving activities such as mindfulness and physically active hobbies can reduce abdominal fat storage, even in the absence of weight loss.

Weight myth no. 7: Society's perception of obesity is fair and helpful

Whether we acknowledge it or not, weight, health and beauty are inextricably linked in our minds. The government often side-steps responsibility for public nutrition education, placing the blame on individuals who are overweight. Concurrently, the media bombards us with unrealistic beauty standards. Our bodies have become a public expression of our discipline, attractiveness, intelligence and even our moral fibre. We're now sold the idea that if you're not quite the model specimen of beauty you deserve to be, there are plenty of cost-effective options to fix this, leading us to starve, sculpt and shape our bodies in pursuit of 'fire' emojis on Instagram.

There are infinite ways to go about it. Just type in #weightloss on any social media platform and you'll be met with fasting pro-tocols, juice cleanses, pills, powders and animal-only or salad-only diets. You can pay thousands of pounds for a 'keto kamp' in the remote Alps, where nobody can hear you cry. Sweat vests, fat-shredding rolling pins and thirty-day ab programmes are all available to enable you to finally become the gorgeous person you've always dreamed of. Welcome to diet culture.

Unfortunately, diet culture also feeds into stereotypical nega-tive beliefs about fat people and their bodies, portraying the overweight as lazy, weak-willed, unattractive, unfit and greedy, which in turn perpetuates weight stigma. Weight stigma is the negative perception of obese people, and the negative attitudes that are directed towards them. This can be in the form of micro-aggressions, such as people tutting or rolling their eyes, or through explicit verbal or physical abuse for someone simply being, well, themselves. This is discrimination which largely stems from ignorance and an entrenched attitude that fatness is entirely a personal responsibility and moral issue, rather than an outcome influenced by a complex mix of biological, socio-environmental and psychological factors.

Even among my peers and other healthcare professionals, it's common to think that shame and fear are good motivators for health improvement,[38] but that's simply not true. An abundance of research shows that when overweight people are subject to weight stigma, they end up eating more. One trial recruited overweight women and subjected them to one of two videos – depicting either weight-stigmatizing or weight-neutral material – after which they were allowed to consume snacks.[39] Because of the emotional stress the footage caused, the women exposed to stigmatizing content ate three times as many calories. This directly challenges the notion that weight stigma has a positive or 'motivating' effect on overweight individuals.

Not only that, but weight stigma leads to poorer food choices, an increased risk of disordered eating, increases in exercise avoidance and worsening substance abuse, such as misusing alcohol.[40] This chronic victimization may even increase death rates in people with obesity. So, while it's important to educate people on the health risks associated with obesity, that does not give anyone the right to belittle, disrespect or bully fat people.

The bottom line: Obesity is inherently harmful to our health, but many people often miss the wood for the trees. Pursuing weight loss shouldn't be about fitting in with societal standards; it should be about improving your health, happiness and longevity so you can truly be the star you deserve to be. Whether you're a healthcare professional, doctor, dietitian, nutritionist, coach or even a friend to someone overweight, the way we communicate about fatness can impact people in more ways than we realize. What may seem like light-hearted banter can often represent the first domino in a long chain of negative consequences.

Weight myth no. 8: It's your fault you're fat

You're just lazy. You sit on your arse all day. Eat a salad! Go to the gym!
Chances are, if you're overweight you've experienced these
insults being thrown at you. They are unkind, stem from an
extremely reductionist viewpoint and demonstrate a lack of
understanding for the complexities and nuance of obesity.

There are countless factors that affect someone's obesity risk,
including biological, environmental and psychological facets. For
example, people with a specific type of mutation in the FTO
gene can't suppress ghrelin (hunger hormone) as efficiently after
a meal, meaning they cannot regulate hunger as well as they
should.[41] For various genetic reasons, identical twins who are
raised apart often end up at similar weights.[42]

Researchers are also now discovering that childhood trauma
plays a significant role in obesity. In addition to leaving deep emotional scars, childhood sexual abuse often turns food into an
obsession for its victims, with many becoming prone to binge-
eating. Others wilfully put on weight to desexualize themselves,
in the hope that what happened to them never recurs. The Nurses'
Health Study of 57,321 adults found that over 10 per cent of
respondents had suffered severe physical or sexual abuse. People
who experienced either form of trauma in childhood had a 90 per
cent increased risk of food addiction.[43] If a child experienced both
physical and sexual assault, their risk of food addiction later in life
was increased by 140 per cent. Women with food addiction were
six BMI units heavier than women without food addiction.

Personal trauma is just one environmental factor that plays a
role in obesity risk; another is geographical location. Did you
know that where you live is one of the biggest predictors for
obesity? Food accessibility and the socio-economic factors that
influence our weight should not be ignored. Around 13.5 million
households in the US contend with food insecurity,[44] meaning

they lack constant access to enough food for an active, healthy lifestyle for all household members. Unsurprisingly, a disproportionate percentage of these people are obese.

I want to give you an example of how utterly ridiculous and obesogenic our food environment is in the UK, from my working life as a doctor. One Friday afternoon, as I stood in a bustling hospital canteen in Birmingham, I found myself face-to-face with an eye-opening realization. Friday in Britain comes with the tradition of fish and chips. This Friday was no exception, and a plate of deep-fried battered fish, a mound of crispy chips and a side of sauce was duly available, all for a modest £2.75. Being wary of oily food, especially when I have to maintain a clear head to attend to my patients, I decided to pair my meal with a small salad pot.

I was hoping that the vibrant, crunchy greens would lend some healthfulness to my lunch and perhaps boost my cognition. But the tiny offering (a handful of lettuce, two cherry tomatoes, three slices of cucumber and some red pepper) cost me a whopping £3. As I stared down at my beige, greasy fish and chips amounting to 2,000 calories, the reality dawned on me. Even armed with the nutritional wisdom I'd gained over the years, guiding patients to limit calorie-rich fried foods, I found myself cornered by limited food choices.

That moment was a stark reminder of the crucial role our food environment plays in our health. Regardless of how high your food IQ may reach, without the means to make healthier choices, that knowledge is virtually powerless. The UK government's recent law mandating restaurants to display calorie counts next to dishes only underscores the issue. Rather than addressing the root problem, it adds another layer of responsibility on the consumer, conveniently deflecting blame away from the government and food manufacturers. Amid increasing poverty, escalating cost of living and soaring fuel prices, the notion of 'just opt for the low-calorie meal to lose weight' sounds preposterous. It detracts from the need for governmental action to enhance our food supply.

So what kind of interventions might help? The changes that would be most meaningful require political clout and determination at every level of government. We've seen this happen in the fossil fuel industry, for example. There have been regulatory interventions including a ban on diesel cars being manufactured after 2035, obliging the leading automotive brands to create affordable electric alternatives. When it comes to nutrition, we've seen it successfully done with the sugar tax, which took a lot of work and coordination behind the scenes across multiple sectors. Following a report from the Scientific Advisory Committee on Nutrition, which recommended a target of 5 per cent dietary energy from free sugars, the UK government challenged the food industry to reduce the sugar content of foods by 20 per cent by 2020.[45] Then, in March 2016, it announced a three-tiered levy on sugary drinks, which was the first soft-drink tax in the world to have multiple tiers and was designed to drive reformulation. Products that contained more than 5–8g of sugar per 100ml were taxed at 18 pence per litre, whereas products with <5g per 100ml were not subject to the tax. The challenge to the food industry to reformulate the nation's favourite soft drinks was accompanied by large public awareness campaigns, as seen in the Change4Life initiative, as well as increased attention to sugar-related harm in the media.[46]

This intervention has largely been successful, with 70 per cent of Britain's soft drinks now containing artificial sweeteners instead of added sugar, to reduce total calories and sugar intake. The same can be said for salt reduction in food. From 2003 to 2018, average salt intake reduced from 9.38g to 8.38g per day as a result of the UK Salt Reduction Strategy.[47] This stepwise reduction of sodium in the food supply over time has contributed to the lowering of stroke and cardiovascular disease mortality in the UK population, and is set to prevent 83,000 cases of ischaemic heart disease and 110,000 premature strokes, and save £1.64 billion in the UK alone by 2050.[48]

The model for real change is there. We have the templates. We have the evidence that it can be done, so it successfully and meaningfully impacts lives. The government just needs to act. The next step is to apply existing policies to other dietary factors that would help combat obesity, such as reducing total calorie intake and saturated fat, while increasing the fibre content of foods. A practical example of this would be to set certain 'healthfulness' criteria for cheap consumable products via tax levies, essentially forcing the food industry to reformulate their products to meet these targets if they want to maintain market share and remain profitable. For instance, instead of a buying a standard chocolate bar for 75p, you could buy a similarly priced, healthier version that contained >5g fibre, <2g saturated fat and was under 150kcal. This would hypothetically score in all three domains and be ranked 'healthfulness rating 3'.

The bottom line: It's important that we start to appreciate some of the nuance surrounding obesity and the social determinants of health and weight. There needs to be major reform in how the government views food policy and obesity if they want to ease the economic burden on healthcare systems and improve people's quality of life. Many factors influencing obesity are not in our control. That being said, we can do our best in the here and now to act on the things we do have control over.

Key takeaways

1. **Fat cells, or adipocytes, play essential roles in survival.** They act as energy banks, help in thermoregulation and produce hormones like leptin and adiponectin that regulate energy intake and insulin resistance. However, excessive adipose tissue can lead to health issues.
2. **Global obesity rates are alarming.** With 13 per cent of people globally and 43 per cent of adults in the US

classified as obese, obesity presents significant physical and mental health challenges, including discomfort and self-esteem issues.

3. **Excess body fat can lead to numerous health problems.** Beyond physical discomfort, excessive fat tissue (especially visceral fat) causes insulin resistance, elevated blood lipids and hypertension, as well as the biochemical products of fat tissue that can release harmful pro-inflammatory and pro-thrombotic chemicals into the bloodstream. This increases the risk of cardiovascular disease, metabolic diseases, cancer and mental health disorders like depression.

4. **Weight loss can improve health.** Studies suggest that even when lifestyle changes do not necessarily promote health, the associated weight loss can still have beneficial effects on health markers. Therefore, while lifestyle changes are crucial, weight loss itself can also contribute to improved health outcomes.

5. **The BMI is useful:** Although the Body Mass Index (BMI) has been criticized for its origins and applicability to diverse populations, it remains a useful tool for predicting body fat percentage and disease risk across populations – when not used in isolation.

6. **The 95 per cent failure rate of diets can be debunked.** The widely perpetuated statistic that 95 per cent of diets fail is based on outdated and contextually limited studies. The definition of 'success' in dieting needs to be redefined as achieving clinically meaningful improvements in health, which can be seen with as little as 5–10 per cent weight loss. These meaningful thresholds have been demonstrated time and time again over many years.

7. **Diet culture and weight stigma cause harm.** Our society's obsession with particular body types has led to

the proliferation of a harmful diet culture and widespread weight stigma. Negative assumptions about obese people, including accusations of laziness and a lack of willpower, are deeply rooted in societal beliefs. Weight stigma is not a motivator for health improvement but leads to adverse health outcomes, including increased caloric intake, poor food choices, disordered eating and substance misuse.

8. **Obesity is complex.** The causes of obesity are multifaceted, and it's erroneous to solely blame an individual for their excess weight. Genetic factors, psychological triggers such as childhood trauma, and the social determinants of health such as geographical location significantly influence an individual's obesity risk.

9. **Food environment and accessibility are important.** Socio-economic and geographic environments significantly influence food choices and obesity risks. With healthier food choices often being more expensive and less accessible, those in poorer households or living in 'food deserts' are disproportionately affected. Government policies often place the responsibility on the consumer, ignoring the larger structural issues at play.

10. **Sustainable weight-loss strategies do exist.** Recognizing the complexity of obesity and understanding the influence of various social determinants of health is crucial. There's a need for systemic reform in food policy and obesity management. While many factors influencing obesity are beyond individual control, there are steps people can take to manage their weight sustainably. These strategies will be outlined in the following chapter.

Weight Loss
Achieving Sustainability

Just eat less and move more, right? Well, the answer is yes . . . but also no.

Hopefully, by now you're aware that the Energy Balance Model (EBM) of obesity, being the scientific consensus, stipulates that the only way to lose weight is to induce a calorie deficit, or to expend more energy than you consume. And it's true that following reductionist pieces of advice like 'eat less, move more' can make it pretty easy to lose 20lb or perhaps even 40lb of weight. Just take your pick out of any of the mainstream fad diets from the first chapter of this book.

It turns out that *sustainable* weight loss isn't as simple as exercising more and consuming less food, however. Sustainable loss is much more complex and multifaceted. Happily, though, we can turn to a hugely helpful study which has shown what habits to employ to lose large amounts of weight *and* keep it off . . . It's called the National Weight Control Registry (NWCR).[1]

The NWCR is the largest weight-loss research study ever run on over 10,000 successful 'dieters' who lost on average 66lb and – crucially – kept it off for more than five and a half years. Eighty per cent of the participants were women, with an average age of forty-five. We also know that 45 per cent of these participants lost the weight on their own, without any guidance, which should give you hope that with nothing but the advice contained in this book, your chances of success are strong. By assessing these women's habits and finding common ground among them, we can pick out the very best strategies to achieve sustainable weight loss.

Eat breakfast every day

Of the successful NWCR dieters, 78 per cent ate breakfast every day. Eating a wholesome breakfast helps regulate appetite across the rest of the day, improves glycaemic function and fatty acid breakdown, burns more calories through the thermic effect of food (TEF), which is the number of calories required to digest and process food, regulates normal circadian fluctuations, as well as aiding general movement (non-exercise activity thermogenesis, or NEAT), exercise habits (exercise activity thermogenesis, or EAT), mental health and energy levels.

Controlled trials show that prioritizing a larger breakfast and a smaller dinner leads to greater levels of weight loss, in some cases *doubling* the effect! There are several reasons why this happens. There appear to be subtle differences in the thermic effect or energy expenditure from a circadian rhythm standpoint later in the day. However, this is marginal at best. The bigger player is that front-loading energy intake likely has positive effects on our general movement and activity levels (NEAT and EAT), as well as benefits for mood and subjective energy or fatigue levels.

In addition, brand-new, tightly controlled research has shown that larger breakfasts are significantly better at suppressing hunger throughout the day, even at subsequent mealtimes.[2] A greater suppression of hunger means less energy intake through food overall. These factors together could explain why many free-living trials (where people are left to their own devices) experience superior weight-loss benefits.

Weigh yourself once a week

Weighing yourself is a way to stay on track for your goals and serves as a regular reminder of the journey you're on. Seventy-five per cent of people who successfully lose large amounts of weight weigh themselves at least once a week. However, if you don't find weighing yourself a positive experience, there are many alternatives, backed by science, like the following:

- Limb or waist measurements (e.g. using a measuring tape around your waist or legs)
- Exercise monitoring (tracking activity levels, cardiovascular fitness or strength, e.g. *Have I managed 10,000 steps today? Does twenty minutes on the treadmill feel easier now? Do I need to increase the weight on my squats?*)
- Calorie counting or food diaries (using apps like MyFitnessPal or a notebook).

It is worth stressing that self-monitoring through regular weighing or calorie counting can be damaging to some people's mental state. If you feel overly anxious or your behaviour regarding weighing yourself becomes obsessive, it may not be the most effective approach for you. While the vast majority of sustainable weight-loss achievers do use a form of self-monitoring, you should reflect on how the process affects you psychologically and realize that it's not mandatory for achieving success.

Watch less than ten hours of TV a week

The national average of time spent watching TV in the US is a huge twenty-eight hours a week.[3] Compare this to the NWCR participants, of whom 62 per cent watched less than ten hours per week, and 36 per cent watched less than five hours per week. Staying sedentary for prolonged periods of time is entirely counterproductive when it comes to managing your weight, not just due to a lack of movement but also the knock-on effects on energy levels, mental health and accompanying eating habits. A meta-analysis of thirteen studies found that binge-watching TV significantly increased the risk of five mental health disorders, in particular stress and anxiety.[4]

Exercise for at least one hour each day

It's no surprise that exercising can help expend more calories, thus making weight loss easier. Hundreds of RCTs show that exercise independently induces modest amounts of weight loss, even without dietary changes.[5] Research also shows that 90 per cent of successful dieters exercise for about one hour per day. However, something that is often overlooked is exercise's ability to improve almost all aspects of health and daily structure. It can provide a sense of fulfilment and instil a secondary wave of energy and motivation midway through the day.

Creating habits and routine is a fundamental part of weight maintenance and healthy living.[6] So even if your exercise routine isn't built to burn a lot of calories, maintaining consistency will positively impact many other aspects of your life, making a weight-loss journey easier to maintain and more gratifying.

Ironically, it's important to note that going 'extra hard' in the gym or trying to burn lots of calories through exercise may not further aid weight loss. The Constrained Energy Model pioneered by Dr Herman Pontzer, associate professor of evolutionary anthropology and global health at Duke University, stipulates that the body adapts to increased physical activity by reducing energy spent on other physiological processes, thus maintaining total energy expenditure within a narrow range.[7] This means that burning more energy from training tends to negatively impact general movement (NEAT) and simultaneously drive up appetite for hyper-palatable foods. Hence why studies like the E-MECHANIC trial demonstrate that around 30 per cent of calories burned from exercise are compensated for through appetite increases and subsequent calorie intake.[8] Therefore higher-intensity or longer exercise sessions don't always mean better results.

So, instead of focusing on the calorie burn from your exercise (and bear in mind that watches, treadmills and waistband monitors are not always accurate), it's more productive to do what you enjoy and can see yourself doing consistently long-term.

Move beyond black-and-white thinking

Being flexible in your dietary choices is often looked at in a negative light. Critics might suggest 'You're just not disciplined enough' or 'You don't want it enough' or ask 'Why are you eating these bad foods?' Ironically, this rigid mindset around food is in fact typical of weight-loss failure, while allowing all foods into your diet is a predictor of weight-loss maintenance.[9] Referring to foods as 'good' or 'bad' is an example of dichotomous or black-and-white thinking. Holding this psychological belief around food predisposes you to poorer health outcomes and weight.

One study of 241 adults found dichotomous beliefs about food impeded the participants' ability to maintain a healthy weight.[10] Other research shows that being all-inclusive with respect to food leads to better weight-loss outcomes,[11] which is supported by a separate study that forced one group to cut out bread – unsurprisingly, they had three times as many dropouts as the control group.[12] It is clear that encouraging strict behaviours around food choices does no one any favours, and could even be harming your physical and mental health. You shouldn't feel bad about that weekend meal out at your favourite restaurant, or your friend's birthday barbecue. Ultimately, it's about balance and long-term habits: one day's slip is not going to make a difference. We know that not all foods are equally nutritious, but understanding that all foods can have a place in a weight-loss journey is important.

Learn about protein and fibre

I'm sure by now you've heard about the importance of protein and fibre for any weight-loss journey. Protein is the most satiating macronutrient and provides the highest thermic effect (20–30 per cent), making it essential in any weight-loss programme. However, it's *not* essential for weight loss per se, as many people easily lose weight on low-protein plant-based diets because they are minimally processed and rich in fibre and whole grains.

Protein is however essential for its ability to preserve muscle mass as you lose weight. Muscle mass is a pillar of longevity and quality of life, because it acts as a metabolic sink for glucose and aids in cardiovascular fitness and bone health – all of which will heavily influence your health in older age.[13] Higher-fibre carbs also have a relatively high thermic effect, sitting at around 20 per cent, are largely unabsorbed by the body, work extremely well to fill you up and provide an abundance of metabolic and gut benefits.

Minimize ultra-processed foods

In one study, healthy adults were given 42g of almonds (30–35 almonds) in their original, whole, raw form, and as a result, they absorbed on average 185kcal. When they were given the exact same quantity of almonds but in the form of almond butter, they absorbed a whopping 274kcal.[14] That's a more than 50 per cent increase in calorie yield, simply due to the processing of that food.

Various studies have demonstrated that food form impacts macronutrient absorption. The absorption of fat from whole nuts is less than from other forms of nuts, suggesting that the chemical bonds between nutrients within food impacts the metabolizable energy of food.[15] A similar phenomenon is seen in a study involving nutrient-identical cheese sandwiches.[16] A processed white bread and cheese sandwich reduced the post-meal energy expenditure (or TEF) by 65 calories, compared to a multigrain version of the same sandwich – meaning that participants burned significantly fewer calories digesting the white bread sandwich.[17] That equates to almost a 50 per cent reduction in TEF, which could drastically reduce how many calories you burn in the day if all your meals are ultra-processed.

This principle also applies to liquid calories in the form of juices, soft drinks, sodas and milkshakes. Sugar-sweetened beverages, also a type of ultra-processed product, have consistently been tied to weight gain because of their calorie density, which is accompanied by minimal satiety effects.[18] To highlight the lack of satiety of ultra-processed foods, when participants were admitted to a research facility for two weeks, they were given diets with *identical* macronutrient compositions – same calories, protein, fibre, sugar, sodium and so on. The sole point of difference between diets was the level of processing of the food. Participants were instructed to eat as little or as much as they wanted, and it was found that the ultra-processed group consumed a whopping 500kcal more per day than the unprocessed group.[19] This lead to 2lb of weight gain, whereas the unprocessed group *lost* 2lb of weight. Just two weeks of following these diets led to a 4lb weight difference between groups!

In short, the more that food is broken down prior to consumption, the less your body must work once it is ingested. Heavily processing and cooking food can lead to an increase in calorie intake via reduced satiety, increased absorption from those foods and a decrease in calorie expenditure, even when nutrient profiles are identical to unprocessed foods.

It is important to avoid liquid calories and prioritize minimally processed whole foods in order to help the energy balance equation to work in your favour.

It's not as simple as counting calories

Calories in, calories out. This simple rubric defines the weight-loss strategy of over a billion people worldwide. While we've established that a calorie deficit is the mechanism by which weight loss occurs, the strategy of calorie counting to achieve said deficit is probably not the wisest. One issue is that people are notoriously bad at calculating their calorie intake;[20] we also tend to overestimate the calories we burn from exercise, sometimes substantially.[21]

I've worked with many patients suffering with eating disorders, who start off on the calorie-counting bandwagon only to become fixated on attributing numbers to all food. When they eat something, all they see are digits, and anything remotely higher than 400kcal is poisonous and toxic . . . even if the dish is a perfectly healthy grilled salmon fillet with avocado and salad. This aligns with the evidence showing that the use of calorie-tracking applications is associated with eating disorder symptomology.[22] One study found that almost 40 per cent of men using a popular tracking app perceived the app as a contributing factor to their disordered eating.[23]

Calorie counting can be a useful tool for some people in helping them stay on track, however due to the difficulty of accurately assessing calorie intake and potential psychological downsides, I believe that educating people on how to implement food strategies that will subconsciously manage levels of intake is generally more productive.

Don't take food labels literally

Food labelling started back in the 1970s, with calorie numbers and sodium content appearing on packets for the reference of those with 'special medical needs'. Fast-forward to today, and of course there are food marketing terms splashed absolutely everywhere; 'gluten-free', 'all-natural', 'GMO-free', 'no added sugar', 'no artificial flavourings' . . . the list goes on. It's not surprising that more than 100 independent studies have demonstrated that many people are confused by modern-day food labels.[24]

Furthermore, they're not always accurate. In the US, for example, nutrition labels are regulated by the Food and Drug Administration (FDA), where a variation of up to 20 per cent in stated calorie amounts is allowed. The UK is not much better. Food labels are regulated by the Food Standards Agency (FSA), yet they don't specify a margin of error, and in many cases they allow food businesses to calculate their own calorie numbers for products. In trials testing dozens of popular snack-food products, bomb calorimetry (the gold standard for assessing caloric value) revealed that some snacks underreported their carbohydrate content by 7.7 per cent.[25] This is also seen in prepared restaurant dishes, where a shrimp and pasta dish stated a count of 250kcal, yet researchers found a count of 319kcal![26] In short, we shouldn't take calorie numbers on packets as literal counts. I don't tend to advise calorie counting to my patients, but if you find it useful as a tool to hold yourself accountable, that's perfectly okay.

Artificial sweeteners are okay

For sweet-toothed individuals, artificially sweetened drinks can help manage cravings without the extra calories of sugar. This supports healthier dietary habits and minimizes added sugars. Moreover, dozens of controlled trials have shown that sweeteners don't seem to increase hunger, provoke cravings or induce obesity.[27] Because of the sustainability they support, in the sense that they can help to suppress sugar cravings, you might even find them superior to water for weight loss, if you're sweet-toothed.

Practise mindful eating

Mindful eating involves paying attention to your food with each passing moment, understanding the purpose of food, eating without judgement, listening to your body and understanding the feeling of satiety. It is the art of being present while you eat. This subject deserves attention as it has been shown to aid weight loss, reduce binge-eating and support good mental health. It's been fundamental in the etiquette of eating in many religions, including the Islamic faith. The Prophet Muhammed (peace be upon him) said: 'No human ever filled a vessel worse than the stomach. Sufficient for any son of Adam are some morsels to keep his back straight. If he likes to have more, then he may fill a third with food, a third with drink, and leave a third for his breath.' This underpins the art of presence surrounding food, with an emphasis on being conscious in the moment and realizing when you're content.

Let's run through some key mindful strategies that can aid a weight-loss journey. First, try to chew at least twenty times per mouthful of food. This helps indigestion and reflux symptoms, and indirectly leads to a reduction in the speed of eating. This is important, because the faster you eat, the more likely you are to overeat.[28] You might find it useful to put your fork down with every bite taken, and only pick it up again once the bite has been thoroughly chewed and swallowed. Similarly, try not to eat and watch TV, or scroll through TikTok on your phone (unless it's my TikTok of course). Aim to eat with no distractions; just you and your plate of food.

Use smaller plates and cutlery

Another practical strategy is to consider your choice of utensils when eating. Plate sizes have been shown to influence our own biases for how filling food will be and how many calories we take in as a result. Larger plates have been linked with larger serving sizes, and unfortunately we have a tendency to want to fill up the empty space on a plate. 'You're not leaving this table until your plate is finished!' was a common refrain at dinner time during my childhood. Even when eighty-five nutrition experts attended an ice cream social, those given the larger bowl served themselves 31 per cent more ice cream without realizing.[29] Smaller spoons have similarly been shown to reduce bite size, eating rate and food intake.[30]

Key takeaways

Obesity is a multifaceted, complicated condition that cannot be boiled down to 'eat less, move more'. Remember this one thing: **your weight does not dictate your worth**, or your value as a person. It is not your fault that you're obese.

There are many things that contribute to obesity that are unfortunately out of our control, however we can only do what we can to lose weight sustainably and improve our health. Here are a few of them:

1. **Behaviours are key.** Successful long-term weight loss is dependent on behaviours, not so much the diet you choose. Hold yourself accountable by taking regular objective measurements (i.e. self-monitor by weighing yourself, keeping a food diary, taking body measurements). Engage in regular exercise, eat breakfast (if it's convenient) and reduce your screen time.

2. **Focus on minimally processed foods.** The closer the food is to its original form, the less 'processed' it is. This will aid in satiety, reduce the calorie density of that food, increase the energy required to digest it and decrease the amount of energy we extract from the food too.

3. **Seek out support.** Find someone to check in on you, and provide advice, support and reminders. Perhaps a gym partner – or arrange a weekly café meet-up with a pal on a similar mission.

4. **Don't be afraid to utilize low-calorie products.** Low- or no-calorie food and drink products are excellent substitutions for the full-sugar versions. They can help in reducing total calories and added sugar intake, and give you a sweet kick that can keep sugar cravings at bay.

5. **Eat consciously and mindfully.** Eat without a distraction. Avoid eating in front of the TV or when working at a desk. Put the fork down between bites. *Chew* your food! These things will help reduce hunger cues, aid satisfaction, and will allow you to understand whether you're actually hungry or just eating because you're distracted.

6. **All chapters in this book and their related topics play a significant role in our ability to regulate weight.** For example, **meal timing** impacts hunger, energy expenditure and sleep quality, which are all crucial to weight management, so make sure to front-load your calories earlier in the day. **Inflammation** can exacerbate metabolic disease and the natural variation in hunger hormones. Disrupted hunger cues can increase energy intake and cravings. **Low mood** or mental health conditions can impact motivation, adherence, increase the likelihood of poorer food choices, cause stress-eating and disrupt your sleep. The health status of our **microbiome** influences energy extraction, expenditure, hunger and mental health. Lastly, all **popular diets** can elicit weight loss by inducing a calorie deficit. Implementing the principles from each chapter will improve your ability to lose weight and keep it off effectively.

PART THREE

New Science

After breaking down prevalent myths surrounding popular diets, inflammation, obesity and weight loss, we stand on the cusp of the future. Welcome to Part Three of *Saturated Facts*, aptly titled 'New Science'. Here, we move away from heavy myth-busting and venture into the pioneering realms of chrononutrition and the importance of meal timing, unearth the mysteries of the gut microbiome, and explore the intricate relationship between diet, depression and dementia. Prepare to be enlightened as we navigate these exciting frontiers, expanding our understanding of nutrition and its far-reaching impact on our health and well-being.

Chrononutrition and Sleep
Time on Your Plate

The concept that what matters is not just *what* you eat but *when* you eat might feel like an entirely new dimension to your understanding of diet and health.[1] In the last chapter, we explored the profound impact of dietary choices on weight management, unearthing the mechanisms behind caloric balance, macronutrient composition and the science of satiety. We examined how adjusting what we put on our plates can tip the scale towards successful weight loss.

However, the story doesn't end with the nutritional composition of our meals. The *timing* of our food consumption plays a compelling role in our health and well-being, including on journeys towards weight loss. Welcome to the world of chrononutrition, a field of study that marries the disciplines of nutrition and chronobiology. It takes into account our internal biological clocks (*chrono* meaning 'time'), which regulate numerous physiological processes – including digestion, metabolism and hormone production. As we delve deeper, we'll uncover how aligning our meal timings with these biological rhythms can not only amplify weight-loss efforts but also improve our overall health. So, let's embark on this journey together, exploring the fascinating interplay of time, food and our bodies.

The medieval Jewish philosopher Maimonides (1135–1204) had a very particular approach to healthy eating. He gave instructions on how to lead a healthy life, and part of those teachings was what, when and how much you should eat. Perhaps his most well-known quote is: 'Eat like a king in the morning, a prince at noon, and a peasant at dinner.' In the past ten years, evidence has emerged showing that meal timing can indeed affect a wide array of physiological processes.

Chrononutrition fact no. 1: The time you eat food makes a difference to health

So why does it matter what time of day we eat? In short, the body struggles to metabolize nutrients at night. Have you ever wondered why or how your body knows to feel tired when it's close to bedtime? Or pondered why, after a lazy day in bed, even though you've slept all day, you never really feel refreshed? This is because humans have evolved to follow a 'diurnal' existence, otherwise known as the sleep/wake cycle or circadian rhythm.

All our internal processes follow a roughly 24-hour cycle. Metabolic processes are optimized in the day, and down-regulate in the night to allow our body time to recover. This works to our advantage, as during daylight hours the cellular functions responsible for homeostasis (our body's ability to stabilize our internal environment) are at their most efficient, in order to allow for any change in the environment. For example, when I'm doing an exhausting thirteen-hour hospital shift, I feel my brain begin to tire and become less efficient nearer the evening, when night falls. This is natural, as during our daily activities our brains need to be switched on so we can think, complete tasks and communicate. A constant stream of energy from glucose and other compounds, as well as 'alert' hormones like cortisol and serotonin, helps us to function. But this process starts to wind down as the day draws to an end.

Our ancestors had an even greater need for this daytime optimization, as often it could mean the literal difference between life and death. The sympathetic nervous system responsible for our 'fight-or-flight' response also needs to work better in the day, so we can act quickly in times of danger. This leads to the release of adrenaline and cortisol, which act to increase our heart rate and glucose output from the liver (hepatic gluconeogenesis). This process gave our ancestors the best chance of successfully escaping a wild animal or beating a threatening opponent, as through it, blood vessels fill with sugar that is ready to be utilized as energy when needed. After the dangerous episode has passed, these mechanisms turn off, allowing the body to return to baseline.

The human body is governed by its circadian rhythms. These rhythms exist because nearly every tissue and organ contains an internal biological clock, which facilitates the circadian cycle. Imagine that inside your body, a factory manager is standing at the top of a production line of tightly packaged boxes of calories. Each box represents energy being directed to various parts of the factory floor, and the individual workers pushing these boxes in different directions represent our metabolic processes and hormones. The manager is observant, glaring down at their employees, telling them when to start or stop. Without supervision, there might be areas of the factory floor not functioning at their best or most efficient. The manager – who represents our circadian 'master clock' – facilitates all operations and ensures they are smooth, timely and without complication. Countless 'peripheral clocks' answer to this one master clock – known as the suprachiasmatic nucleus (SCN), a highly specialized part of the hypothalamus in the brain which receives signals directly from the eyes. To maintain homeostasis, the body's peripheral clocks synchronize themselves to the SCN. Many functions of metabolism and digestion follow a roughly 24-hour cycle based on cycles of light and dark.

One example of a peripheral clock is the digestive system. A broad range of vital functions within the digestive system display circadian variations. For instance, the mouth produces saliva to aid digestion and the passage of food down the oesophagus. We now know that the volume of saliva produced is increased during daylight hours. Saliva contains key enzymes, such as amylase, which help break carbohydrates down into glucose. This is why if you chew a savoury cracker for a long time, you'll eventually taste the hidden sweetness within.

Another example of how our digestive tract is optimized in the day is through the movement of food. Gastric emptying rates (which means the speed at which food exits our stomach) are shorter in the daytime, and peristalsis in the digestive tract (muscular contractions that move food through the gut) are also linked to a circadian cycle. The opposite is demonstrated in the evening, as we see a reduction in movement of food through the large bowel during sleep.[2]

Our feelings of hunger and satiety, while complex, are linked to two hormones named ghrelin and leptin. Ghrelin is typically referred to as the 'hunger hormone', while leptin is the 'fullness hormone'. These hormones synchronize to our usual meal timing, so people who typically eat breakfast will feel hungry upon waking. This is also seen in those who practise intermittent fasting or observe the holy month of Ramadan. The first few days of fasting are notoriously difficult, as your digestive system is used to you waking up and eating. However, after a few days, your body gets the message and fasting becomes easier. This is why people no longer feel hungry after a few days of skipping breakfast.

Now that we've established a basic understanding of our body's circadian rhythms and how they relate to digestion, let's look at what happens when we eat at different times of the day.

Chrononutrition fact no. 2: The harmful effects of a late dinner

A useful scenario to look at when considering this idea is what happens when you eat a heavy meal at night, compared to earlier in the day. Those who habitually eat at night are seen in observational studies to have an increased risk of metabolic conditions such as type 2 diabetes and cardiovascular disease. This is becoming more commonplace in Western countries – people in the US often consume around a third of their calories after 6 p.m., and the UK has seen a trend in increasing energy intakes in the afternoon and evening, too.[3] Current dietary habits show that we consume up to 40 per cent of our energy intake during the night. But what is happening when we eat later in the day?

Our body is not as capable at regulating our blood sugar levels closer to our 'circadian night' – or within a few hours of the time we normally sleep. Throughout evolutionary history, we've not had to regulate blood sugar levels as aggressively throughout the day as we do now, because in earlier times we would usually have had less immediate access to food. Gone are the days when you'd have to stalk a small mammal for hours, hunt it, kill it and prepare it before having your first bite. With modern-day technologies, supply chains and distribution, food is now easily accessible to most people in the Western world at any time of day. Every major road now has either a supermarket or a convenience store where you can pick up all of your favourite treats. This is the only time period in human existence when we can press a button and, fifteen minutes later, a freshly made katsu curry is on the doorstep.

One research study exploring this took twenty healthy volunteers with a fixed bedtime of 11 p.m. They were given a dinner consisting of exactly the same food either at 6 p.m. or 10 p.m. The group that consumed dinner at 10 p.m. had a higher postprandial glucose peak, meaning their glucose rose to higher levels in response to their food intake. This means a longer period of time spent with higher blood glucose, which over time can damage cells. The group also had lower levels of dietary fatty-acid oxidation (the breakdown of fats in the meal), indicating an inefficiency in food metabolization and increased cortisol levels, suggesting a disruption in hormonal regulation.[4] These differences show that consuming food later in the day negatively impacts various metabolic processes important for optimal health. The researchers concluded that these metabolic effects could promote obesity if they were to occur chronically.

Similar findings were seen in a randomized crossover trial which took place over two weeks.[5] Eleven healthy women were instructed to consume a 200kcal snack, comprising mainly fats and carbs, every day for thirteen days either at 10 a.m. or at 11 p.m. On day 14, they entered a respiratory chamber and their energy metabolism was measured for twenty-three hours. The researchers found that, relative to daytime snacking, night-time snacking significantly decreased fat oxidation and increased total and low-density lipoprotein (LDL) cholesterol. LDL cholesterol is typically referred to as 'bad cholesterol', as it carries cholesterol to your arteries where it can be deposited, contributing to plaque formation. The researchers discovered that changing the time of the small snack increased cholesterol by 9mg/dL and LDL by 7mg/dL. In units more familiar to the UK, shifting the time of that small snack to night equated to a cholesterol increase of about 0.6mmol/L (<5mmol/L is a healthy level). Now, if that small snack turned into the kind of large evening meal so many adults in the Western world eat regularly, this blood lipid difference would be much more detrimental.

Research experiments on rodents have shown how meal timing can alter how certain cholesterol-converting enzymes are expressed, which leads to an increase in cholesterol synthesis.[6] As LDL cholesterol plays a causal role in cardiovascular disease,[7] this adds to the weight of evidence suggesting that habitual night-time eating increases the risk of cardiovascular disease. These findings have been supported by a recent analysis of ten controlled studies – which concluded that people who habitually eat at night have poorer post-prandial glucose tolerance.[8]

The bottom line: Eating food late in the day negatively affects various metabolic processes important for optimal health. Harmful effects include: poorer glucose tolerance, reduced ability to metabolize fats, and an increase in cortisol levels and LDL cholesterol. Therefore, try to avoid large meals within a few hours of your normal sleep time.

Chrononutrition fact no. 3: Post-meal glucose regulation and the effects of night eating

So why does habitual night-time eating lead to a poorer postprandial glucose tolerance? When we eat, we break down and digest food, which raises our blood sugar levels. The body responds by releasing a surge of the hormone insulin from the pancreas to lower that elevated sugar level. Insulin acts by shuttling the sugar in our blood back into the liver and muscles to be stored as glycogen, or turned into fatty acids to be stored as adipose tissue throughout our body. This is why it's often referred to as a 'storage hormone', because it stores excess energy and saves it for when it's needed.

The amount of insulin your body releases is related to the composition of the meal. Carbohydrate-rich foods are made up of glucose molecules bound together. Naturally, these foods, like rice and pasta, will cause the biggest surge in blood sugar and therefore insulin, whereas those with healthy fats like avocados or protein-rich foods cause a smaller rise. This is why people living with type 1 diabetes have to manually carb count to calculate how much insulin they need, as their pancreas isn't doing it automatically.

Sometimes this insulin surge is too much for the food that was ingested and can lead to a state called postprandial or reactive hypoglycaemia, where blood glucose levels temporarily fall below the normal range within a few hours of eating. This is typically due to an underlying condition such as insulin resistance or type

2 diabetes, gastrointestinal issues or hormone deficiencies, but is also common in overweight people and in meals that are heavy in refined sugars.[9] The body functions best in a very tightly controlled environment. So this temporary drop in blood sugar activates several homeostatic responses by the body in an attempt to restore normal bodily function.

One way in which the body attempts to restore sugar levels is to release hormones such as cortisol and adrenaline, which play a role in blood glucose control as previously described. Cortisol can act to increase cravings for hyper-palatable foods that are rich in both sugars and fats. Temporarily low blood sugar can also induce lethargy or fatigue, which could psychologically sway you into eating more food. Night-time eating leads to worsening regulation of these metabolic pathways, potentially leading us to consume more high-sugar and fatty foods. To combat our inefficiency in regulating blood sugar, we should try to avoid carbohydrate-heavy meals in the evenings and prioritize adding fibre and dietary protein to our dinner. This will help minimize the amount of time spent with abnormally high blood glucose, therefore protecting your blood vessels and cells over the long run.

Chrononutrition fact no. 4: How meal timing affects the thermic effect of food

The energy required to digest, process and absorb the food we eat is called the thermic effect of food (TEF). Fats have a TEF of 0–3 per cent, carbohydrates 5–10 per cent and protein a whopping 20–30 per cent.[10] This means that if you were to consume 100kcal of pure chicken breast, your body would spend up to 30 of those calories processing it, thus netting only 70 calories. So logically, eating more protein-rich foods results in a higher energy expenditure, something that most active people would desire. Simply increasing the percentage of protein in your diet without increasing total calories has been shown to increase energy expenditure by 100–200 calories per day. How does this relate to meal timing, you ask? There's evidence that the thermic effect of food is up to 50 per cent lower in the night, resulting in a higher net intake of calories with those meals.[11] If you normally expend 100 calories on digestion in the morning, the same meal might only use 50 calories on digestion at night.*[12]

The human body loves routine. It thrives on metabolic regularity and order. This is why the regularity of when we eat our meals seems to affect TEF as well. Studies have found that having an irregular eating schedule by changing your meal timing and frequency has a detrimental effect on your TEF, resulting in a net increase in calories.[13]

It is therefore important to eat on a more regular schedule and introduce more protein earlier in the day, to synchronize our peripheral biological clocks (e.g. the digestive system) with the master clock (SCN) in order to optimize metabolic function and therefore overall health. Now we've seen some of the direct physiological effects of eating late at night, let's explore some of the indirect negative effects on our health.

---

* Interestingly, this reduction in calories burned post-evening meal may not necessarily be down to a reduced thermic effect itself, but rather our basal metabolic rate simply being lower during the night-time. This has been demonstrated in a brand-new study that tested fourteen overweight individuals at a clinical research unit. The subjects ate breakfast, lunch and dinner at the facility and their basal metabolism and thermic effect were calculated. Researchers found that when they factored in the reduction in metabolism during the evening, the thermic effect from those meals actually stayed the same. So, although the overall calories expended were reduced later in the day, resting metabolism is what constituted that reduction and not the thermic effect of food. What we can conclude is that our body expends fewer calories later in the day. Whether that's from TEF or simply a reduction in basal metabolic rate is an academic point at best.

Chrononutrition fact no. 5: Late eating decreases daytime energy

If you consistently consume a large proportion of your daily calories at night (within a few hours of your typical bedtime = circadian night), you're at risk of not adequately fuelling your body in the day when you're awake. This means you won't be as energized or move around as much.

Think about a time when you didn't eat lunch or dinner. Were you as keen to go for a walk, do your chores – or even socialize for that matter? Probably not. This is because your body subconsciously tells you to conserve energy by not moving around as much, making you feel lazier. So not only will your general movement be decreased, but your exercise intensity and duration will likely suffer as well. A meta-analysis of thirty-seven controlled studies showed that for exercise sessions lasting longer than sixty minutes, eating something prior to that workout saw improved exercise performance and capacity in the majority of studies analysed.[14]

Any movement that is dedicated to structured exercise is referred to as exercise activity thermogenesis (EAT), while general movement and fidgeting in the day are non-exercise activity thermogenesis (NEAT); this includes things like doing chores, commuting to and from work, or even scratching your head while seated at your desk. Ensuring adequate calorie intake early in the day will likely have positive effects in terms of both EAT and NEAT and how much energy you expend across a 24-hour period.

Chrononutrition fact no. 6: Eating before bed impacts sleep and mood

Eating close to your bedtime can negatively impact your sleep and mood.[15] This is because when we eat late at night, the muscles and organs that digest and metabolize food are forced to work when they should be resting. This goes against our circadian rhythm and can delay our ability to fall asleep, thus hindering the descent into the deep sleep phase.

Not only does it delay our sleep time, it can disrupt intermittent portions of our sleep as well. Not to mention the vicious cycle that could be initiated: eating at night affects sleep, poorer sleep increases night-time cravings, and more food at night further impacts sleep. Deep sleep is the most restful stage of the sleep cycle and is required to feel refreshed and energized the next day. Adequate sleep duration and quality are an essential part of healthy metabolic function and weight management, which we will explore later in this chapter. Sleep deprivation leads to increased appetite (especially for hyper-palatable foods), stress, lower energy levels, influences poor dietary choices and lowers your resting metabolic rate.

The overwhelming amount of observational evidence across tens of thousands of individuals shows that habitual night-eating puts you at a higher risk of cardiometabolic disorders such as cardiovascular disease, type 2 diabetes and obesity, and leads to reduced success in weight-loss trials. The research shows that for people who are actively trying to lose weight, or make some dietary changes, those who eat a significant proportion of calories at night are at a much higher risk of failing the task they set out for themselves.[16] This is likely due to heightened cravings at night, poorer sleep quality and reduced EAT and NEAT, as well as more complex psychological issues such as boredom or emotional eating.

Chrononutrition fact no. 7:
Meal timing can affect your weight

Now we understand the mechanisms by which eating a large proportion of calories towards the end of the day can alter various metabolic processes and have a negative impact on our health. It then becomes clear how these factors can shift the 'calories in vs calories out' equation against us, leading to weight gain.

Several controlled studies show that eating at night influences a person's weight negatively. In a recent study, researchers took eighty-two women and split them into two weight-loss groups for a duration of twelve weeks. Both groups were put on around a 500kcal deficit diet, with the only difference being the time at which they had their dinner: 7.30 p.m. vs 10.30 p.m. Researchers found that the early dinner group lost an average of 2.5kg more than the late dinner group, and had improved blood lipids and insulin sensitivity (your body's ability to utilize insulin and therefore regulate blood sugar).[17] That's an extra ½lb of weight loss per week simply by changing the time at which they had dinner!

This kind of investigation has been replicated several times. A similar study found that the group that had breakfast as their largest meal lost 5kg more than the group that consumed a heavy dinner. This was despite both groups being prescribed the same 1400kcal per day.[18] In a different study, participants were put onto a low-calorie fixed Mediterranean diet for three months.[19] The researchers evaluated the differences in health markers by changing the distribution of calories throughout the day. Group 1 had 70 per cent of their calories at breakfast, while group 2 had 55 per cent at breakfast. Both groups had improved health outcomes, but group 1 – with the larger breakfast – lost 25 per cent more weight, 50 per cent more fat, an extra inch off of their waists and had greater improvements in insulin sensitivity. Finally, a brand-new randomized control trial demonstrated that those who front-loaded their calories had less daily subjective hunger and appetite, despite both groups consuming the same calories.[20]

To be clear, I'm not suggesting that the solution is simply to add breakfast to your day. If you're used to skipping breakfast and having a substantial lunch and dinner, adding an omelette and toast for breakfast will likely increase or maintain your overall calories for the day.[21]

The bottom line: The overarching theme to take away from this chapter is that shifting the proportion of your calories earlier, or prioritizing your meals in the daylight hours, better aligns with our circadian biology and can positively impact cardiovascular and metabolic health and weight-loss outcomes. So, although the total amount and types of food you eat are the ultimate factor in your cardiometabolic risk and whether you gain or lose weight, we shouldn't ignore the significant role that meal timing and eating in unison with our circadian rhythm have on our overall health. This nicely ties into what is arguably the most important regulator of our circadian biology: sleep.

The importance of sleep

When was the last time you woke up feeling refreshed, energetic and not needing a caffeine boost to get you through the day? If you struggle to answer this question, then know you're not alone. While getting seven to nine hours per night is recommended, around 30 per cent of all adults report sleeping for less than six hours per night;[22] 35 per cent of Americans report sleeping less than seven hours per night, and almost half of all Americans say they feel sleepy between three and seven days per week. Meanwhile, nearly a quarter of adults in the UK manage no more than five hours of sleep, and two-thirds of all adults throughout the developed world fail to meet the eight hours of recommended sleep per night. Inadequate sleep is linked to seven of the fifteen leading causes of death in the US, including cardiovascular disease, cancer, cerebrovascular disease, diabetes, accidents, septicaemia and hypertension.[23]

I used to think that sleep was an entirely separate strand when it came to our health, alongside our food choices and exercise habits. But in fact, it is increasingly clear that it represents the very foundation of our health and well-being. Without good-quality sleep, our dietary and exercise habits take a massive hit. Regular good-quality sleep is the single biggest component of our internal clock, so it makes complete sense that if our sleep is poor, we disrupt the dozens of homeostatic mechanisms needed for health regulation. A good night's sleep empowers the body to recover and lets us wake up refreshed and ready to take on the world. Unfortunately, inadequate sleep is particularly prevalent across the globe. So much so that the World Health Organization has declared a 'global epidemic of sleeplessness'.

Sleep is usually one of the first things people are willing to forgo when they feel pressed for time. This mindset often stems from 'hustle culture' and manifests itself in those who parrot the line 'I'll sleep when I'm dead'. A common thought process is that sleep is a luxury, and daily chores or work should be prioritized over it. Sadly, humans are the only species that will purposefully deprive themselves of sleep without a valid upside. I am personally guilty of this. During the writing of this book I willingly allowed myself to chip away at my precious snooze time for the sake of staring at my laptop screen, struggling to find my next sentence. Terrible, right? And you too might be reading this at an unearthly hour.

We live our lives thinking that the benefits of limiting the hours we sleep outweigh the costs. Many of the downsides of poor sleep go unnoticed and accumulate over a long period of time. Inadequate sleep increases the risk of pretty much all of the chronic lifestyle diseases we're focusing on in this book: cardiovascular disease, type 2 diabetes, obesity and even depression and cancer. I strongly believe that getting enough high-quality sleep is as important to well-being as nutrition and exercise are.

Several large population studies have shown that poor sleep is strongly linked to an increased risk of cardiovascular disease,[24] sometimes with an increase in risk as high as 200 per cent! To understand why poor sleep increases our risk of cardiovascular disease, think of poor sleep as a state of metabolic stress. When the body is stressed, it initiates the inflammatory response, and multiple studies show that people who sleep poorly have increased inflammatory markers in the blood.[25] Poor sleep also leads to a poorer glucose tolerance, which means more time spent with a higher blood glucose.[26] To really put the nail in the coffin, high blood pressure is another bodily response from this state of stress.[27]

All of these factors can damage the lining of the coronary arteries – which, over time, leads to calcification and plaque formation. And when plaque builds up in the arteries, it reduces blood flow to the heart and can even rupture and throw off a clot, causing a heart attack or stroke. These processes are all forms of cardiovascular disease.

But how does poor sleep lead to worsening glucose tolerance? *In vitro* studies have shown that cells from individuals who were forcibly sleep-deprived to just 4.5 hours of sleep for four days became unresponsive to insulin.[28] This meant that their blood sugar stayed high for longer periods of time, and this is one reason why people who are lacking in good-quality sleep have a significantly increased risk of type 2 diabetes.[29] Poor sleep not only changes our bodies' ability to utilize glucose, it also impacts various hormones and brain centres that dictate appetite and food choices.

Less sleep, more weight: hormones and hunger

The reasons behind the recent sharp increase in obesity rates are heavily debated. The rise in consumption of ultra-processed foods and a reduction in daily movement are valid components in this equation, but they are not the only contributing factors. Did you know that regularly sleeping for less than six hours increases your risk of being obese by 55 per cent?[30] Poor sleep contributes in many different ways to weight gain. To understand how a lack of sleep contributes to weight gain, let's first explore what happens to our hunger and fullness hormones when we sleep poorly.

The two main hunger hormones are ghrelin and leptin. Ghrelin is the most commonly known, as it triggers the strong sensation of hunger shortly before eating food or when you've missed a meal. When ghrelin levels increase, so does your appetite. Leptin on the other hand plays a role in many energetic processes, but also signals a sense of fullness. When leptin levels are high, this suppresses your appetite and the desire to eat fades.

A lack of sleep directly affects the levels of these hormones. One study took a cohort of normal-weighted, healthy men and tested them across two sets of two nights' sleep.[31] Researchers compared the effects of ten and four hours of sleep on metabolic parameters. They found that after the nights of just four hours of sleep, the test subjects were significantly hungrier the next day. This is thought to be due to a large drop in their leptin levels (the fullness hormone), at the same time as a sharp rise in their ghrelin levels (the hunger hormone). This was the case despite the identical amount of food being consumed on both occasions. These hormonal changes in response to a single (or row) of sleepless nights have been replicated several times.[32]

But ghrelin and leptin aren't the only hormones that a lack of sleep affects. During a stressful situation, mammals' brains respond by activating something called the hypothalamic–pituitary–adrenal (HPA) axis. This involves three main centres of the body: the hypothalamus and the pituitary gland, located in the brain, and the adrenal glands that lie on top of the kidneys. This triad controls the body's reactions to stress and regulates various bodily processes involved in digestion, immunity, mood and energy usage. This matters because evidence has shown that chronic sleep deprivation causes a disruption to the biological stress response.[33] The disturbance can increase our appetite, particularly for delicious 'naughty' foods. Furthermore, poor sleep triggers the adrenal glands to produce cortisol, and higher baseline cortisol levels are a strong predictor of future weight gain.[34]

These are some of the ways in which poor sleep works against us, and is likely why studies have found that people eat almost 400kcal more when they are sleep-deprived than when they are sufficiently rested.*[35]

---

* Regarding sleep and appetite hormones, it appears that the research is mixed. We know with high confidence that people who are sleep-deprived eat more calories on average and feel a lot hungrier. The key word being 'feel'. A meta-analysis of forty-one randomized controlled trials testing the metabolic differences between normal sleep and sleep restriction in healthy adults found that people consume on average 253 calories more when sleep-restricted. They also found their subjective hunger was significantly higher, participants' weight increased, insulin sensitivity decreased, and brain activity involved in the food reward pathway and cognitive control were heightened. This suggests that hyper-palatable foods that we would class as 'yummy' treats, like cakes and desserts, would be more pleasurable and desirable. However, the surprising finding was that across all of the studies analysed, there was no significant difference in mean leptin or ghrelin levels. So, although there doesn't seem to be a consensus regarding changes in the main appetite hormones, *something* on top of brain activity changes is driving people to eat more when sleep-deprived. Most health books would conclude that sleep causes a disruption in ghrelin and leptin appetite cues; the truth is, research hasn't quite figured it out thus far. Perhaps additional hormonal changes are responsible. Complicated interactions exist between other appetite hormones such as peptide YY, GLP-1, neuropeptide Y and cholecystokinin. There's also some evidence showing that sleep deprivation activates the endocannabinoid system, which may play a key role in hedonic pathways involved in modulating appetite and food intake. These could be appropriate research avenues for the future to determine what exactly is causing this sharp rise in subjective hunger and increased calorie intake.

Tips for better-quality sleep

- **Have a structured exercise routine.** A meta-analysis of thirty-four studies found that regular exercise (not too close to bedtime) improves your sleep quality and duration.[36] This relationship is bi-directional, meaning that improved sleep quality also positively impacts exercise performance. It's a win-win!

- **Create sleep hygiene practices** to aid your body in feeling sleepy. These might include a regular sleeping schedule (going to bed and waking up at the same time); keeping your room nice and cool (we sleep better in cooler temperatures); having a downtime ritual before bed (doing the same 2–3 things before you sleep, e.g. night-time bathroom routine, mindfulness, reading a book for ten minutes, etc.); avoiding time on your phone thirty minutes before bed.

- **Get some sunlight in the morning**, within thirty minutes of waking. Pull the curtains back, step outside. The visual stimulus of daylight is the key regulator of our circadian rhythm. If you don't activate the main stimulus, you can't hope to efficiently regulate all other metabolic processes we've discussed that fall under circadian biology.

- **Avoid large meals close to bedtime.** Consuming large amounts of food or fluid can cause digestive discomfort or force you to urinate in the night. Studies show it can negatively impact your sleep quality due to your body working hard to digest the food rather than focusing on recovery and repair.[37]

The graveyard shift

Given the importance of circadian biology on our overall health and well-being, it shouldn't surprise you that shift workers, who tend to experience disrupted sleep patterns, are at a far greater risk of all the chronic lifestyle diseases mentioned in this chapter.*

As we've previously explored, eating in a manner that contradicts our circadian rhythm leads to decreased glucose tolerance, reduced fatty-acid oxidation, an increase in blood lipids and the biological stress response, and a reduced thermic effect of food. As a hospital doctor I know first-hand about the stresses and struggles of night-shift work. I realize that it's incredibly difficult for many, but what can shift workers do to help mitigate the health risks? Although there aren't many studies directly testing different nutritional strategies to help minimize some of these disturbances during shift work, we can make educated suggestions.

To optimize your health and well-being while working night shifts, one sensible approach is to reduce your intake of carbohydrate- and fat-rich foods during the night, since our bodies metabolize these nutrients less effectively during twilight hours. Instead, focus on consuming high-protein snacks and meals. Try to keep your eating schedule as similar as possible to your daytime routine, as the thermic effect of food is improved when meal timings are consistent. For example, if you typically have dinner at 7.30 p.m. and breakfast at 7.30 a.m., aim to eat around these times even if you're working an 8–8 shift through the night. You

---

Several comprehensive reviews have been recently published in journals such as the *British Medical Journal* (PMID: 34473048), showing that shift workers are at an increased risk of many diseases and cancers, including ones we haven't yet discussed, such as myocardial infarctions (heart attacks) and prostate cancer.

may want to have a small, high-protein snack in the middle of your shift to keep your energy levels up. It's also advisable to avoid eating during the 'danger zone' (the mid-portion of the night, around 1–4 a.m.) when our metabolic processes are least efficient.

You could also consider using blue-light-blocking glasses during your commute home from work to help regulate your body's sleep–wake cycle. These prevent certain wavelengths of light from entering your eyes and can help you feel sleepy, and fall asleep faster. Additionally, it's best to avoid consuming caffeine later in your shift, as it has a long half-life and may interfere with your ability to get high-quality sleep after work. By implementing these strategies, you can help mitigate the effects on your health and well-being of working night shifts.

The field of chrononutrition is a new and exciting one, and it's allowed us further insight into the importance of structuring our mealtimes to align with our circadian rhythm. Not only are the types of foods we eat important for overall health and for reducing our risk of disease, but *when* we eat seems to play an important role too. Naturally, our circadian rhythm is structured around the sleep–wake cycle, so make sure to prioritize sleep quality as well.

Key takeaways

1. **Consume the majority of your calories in the morning and afternoon.** This aids metabolic functioning, general movement, appetite regulation, exercise performance, evening cravings and sleep quality, all of which decrease your risk of disease.
2. **Try to stick to a regular eating schedule,** where the times and frequency of meals are the same, allowing

your circadian rhythm to build routine and function optimally.

3. **Avoid heavy and calorific meals close to bedtime** (especially those rich in carbohydrates or fats). They can negatively impact metabolic processes and indirectly ruin your sleep.

4. **Stick to low-calorie, protein-rich meals outside the 'danger zone'** (1–4 a.m.) if you're a shift worker who needs to eat during the night.

5. **Sleep 7–9 hours per night.** This should be high on your list of priorities! A good night's sleep will provide the foundation for all pillars of health and cannot be emphasized enough. The encouraging news is that getting enough sleep will help you to control your food choices and, indirectly, your body weight. See page 118 for some key tips to improve your sleep quality.

The Gut Microbiome

Man's Best Friend(s)

Following our exploration of the fascinating domain of chrono-nutrition, we now embark on a journey to an equally captivating world within us: our gut microbiome. As we transition into this new realm, we'll see that our relationship with time can also directly influence this complex ecosystem thriving in our digestive tract.

Our gut microbiome is a bustling metropolis of trillions of microbes encompassing bacteria, viruses, fungi and many other microorganisms that call our digestive system home. Just like the tick of the biological clock in chrononutrition, these microbial communities influence and are influenced by our diets, lifestyle choices and even the rhythms of our daily lives. In this chapter we'll explore how this microbial community plays a significant role in digestion, immune function and even our mood. Unravelling the intricate relationship between the gut microbiome and our health will add another layer to our understanding of nutrition's complexity and interconnectedness. We'll learn how nurturing these tiny inhabitants can have far-reaching implications on our health and wellness journey, including our weight management efforts and overall metabolic health.

Every day, we share our food with our best friend. She knows what we like and dislike, she travels with us, we provide a roof over her head and food on her plate, she has evolved with us and we cannot live without her. I'm not referring to the family pet, but something millions of times smaller and invisible to the naked eye. I mean the microbiome: primitive forms of life called microbes that are too small to be seen or felt, often stigmatized for being a source of 'filth' on animals or dirty clothes. They are wildly misunderstood.

Our bodies contain trillions of them, comprising around a quarter of our total number of cells and weighing a whopping 5lb inside our gut, where the majority reside.[1] For many, the idea of the microbiome conjures images of *E. coli*-infested takeaways and uncooked chicken riddled with *Salmonella*, yet it's so much more than that. For a long time, the scientific community considered microbes obsolete, believing they couldn't influence our health in a meaningful way. But it was very wrong.

An entire ecosystem of trillions of bacteria exists within our mouths, guts and skin. This extended genome housed within us is slowly taking the spotlight as a pivotal factor in pretty much all aspects of human health, from immunity and brain function to weight management and cardiometabolic health. The truth is, our understanding of this field of research is embryonic, but what we do know is that dietary factors can significantly influence the composition and 'health' of our gut microbiota.[2] The trendy 'gut health' wave is filled with hyperbole and unscientific extrapolations of mediocre data – from probiotics being hailed as a fix-all solution to the idea that you need to 'cleanse' your gut for optimal health – so in this chapter we will analyse what we do know, debunk some common gut-health myths, and assess the role of the microbiome in human health and how diet impacts this relationship.

Microbiome myth no. 1:
Probiotic supplements will fix your gut issues

Walk into any supermarket and you will likely find more than a few probiotic products allegedly containing beneficial bacteria that will fix your life's problems. A probiotic is defined as live bacteria that positively benefit the host. Typical claims for their benefits include relieving constipation, aiding weight loss and even curing depression. Increasing popularity over the past ten years means shoppers can now acquire probiotic capsules, pills, juices, drinks, cereals, cookies, snack bars and even cosmetics.

An objective assessment of the science underlying microbe-based treatments reveals that most of the health claims are pure hype. There is no evidence to suggest that people with normal gastrointestinal tracts can benefit from taking probiotics. However, there is some benefit for specific groups: a 2014 review by Cochrane (an independent network of experts who serve as rigorous arbiters of medical research) found that probiotics can be particularly useful in neonatal intensive care units.[3] The addition of beneficial bacteria to a nutritional regimen seems to significantly reduce the likelihood of developing necrotizing enterocolitis, a devastating, poorly understood and often fatal gut disease that causes the bowel to become inflamed and die. Up to a third of preterm infants die with this condition, yet the effectiveness of probiotics actually increases when the baby is premature. Leading experts believe this disease arises from an opportunistic infection in the developing gut of an infant. When the gut inflammation becomes too much, it ruptures and floods the abdominal cavity with dangerous microbes. Treatment involves surgery to remove the dead bowel and internally sterilize the body, while providing antibiotics and food via drips. But unless you're a preterm baby, taking regular probiotics is not likely to be of major benefit to your health.

However, probiotics do also seem to benefit some sufferers of irritable bowel syndrome. A review of more than ten clinical trials found that probiotics helped to relieve the symptoms of IBS in a proportion of people.[4] For example, one study of sixty IBS sufferers found that 47 per cent of them noted improvements in their symptoms after taking a specific probiotic daily for four weeks.[5] The reasons for this are largely unknown, with some speculation surrounding probiotics' ability to inhibit the growth of certain harmful microbes. However, the effectiveness of probiotics seems to be strain-specific and varies widely. Furthermore, not all studies have found a benefit, and many trials have limitations such as small sample sizes or short durations. The American Gastroenterological Association has recommended against the use of probiotics for most gastrointestinal conditions, including irritable bowel syndrome, due to a lack of clear evidence. They emphasize that while probiotics are generally safe for healthy individuals, they are not free from side effects and are often expensive. Therefore, while individuals with IBS may choose to experiment with probiotics, it's important to focus on a broader management strategy that includes dietary modifications, stress management and medication as needed.

Commercially manufactured probiotics generally do very little because manufacturers often select bacterial strains that are easy to grow in large numbers over ones which are adapted to the human gut. Typical examples include strains of *Bifidobacterium* or *Lactobacillus* (found in many yoghurts and pills), many of which cannot survive the highly acidic stomach. Even if some do manage to survive and propagate in the intestine, their numbers are insufficient to significantly change our bacterial composition. The human gut contains trillions upon trillions of bacteria, whereas a typical microbe-filled pill has about 100–500 million (0.00001 per cent of our gut microbes).

A team of scientists from the University of Copenhagen published a meta-analysis of seven controlled trials assessing whether biscuit, milk-based or capsule probiotics change the diversity of bacteria in faecal samples in healthy people.[6] They assessed changes in the diversity, number and distribution of bacteria within the faeces. Only one study of thirty-four healthy volunteers saw a change in diversity between samples compared to the placebo. And even then, there was no indication that the said change improved health in any way.

The bottom line: Probiotics aren't particularly useful for most healthy people. Drinking a probiotic supplement is akin to putting a drop of hot water in a water bottle and expecting it to start steaming. Most people will obtain a negligible difference in their gut health from probiotics, though if you are suffering from IBS, certain probiotic products may provide some help depending on the strain. If you do want to try probiotics, try experimenting with one for a few weeks while keeping a symptom diary. The only real damage commercially available probiotic supplements can do is to your wallet.

If you want to see certain improvements in gut health and function, swap the pills, powders and drinks for *dietary* probiotics. These include fermented foods such as yoghurt, milk, sauerkraut, sourdough bread, kefir and a variety of cheeses.

Microbiome myth no. 2: You're probably infested with worms

Yes, you heard me correctly. There are people selling parasitic cleanses online. According to some commentators, *most* of us are infested with live worms inside our guts that are responsible for chronic disease and are the root cause of all illness. Some of the health claims I get tagged in online are so ridiculous I don't even think they warrant discussion, but even though this one is absurd, I do want to touch on it briefly.

Parasites are organisms that live off their 'hosts' in order to survive. The major sources of transmission for parasitic infections stem from tropical climates, poor hygiene, lack of access to clean water, and contaminated food, soil and blood. Some parasitic infections can be asymptomatic, such as that of the *Trypanosoma cruzi* parasite, with which 95 per cent of people in the acute phase show no signs of illness,[7] but if you have an intestinal parasite the likelihood is you will be extremely ill. I'm talking abdominal pain, rapid weight loss, vomiting, nausea, bloating and even bleeding or mucus from the back passage.[8] If you have these symptoms and you're concerned it's a parasite, go to the hospital immediately.

The bottom line: If you're at home, feeling well enough to watch videos online telling you you're infested with parasites . . . then you're not infested with parasites.

Microbiome myth no. 3: Food sensitivity tests are useful

You might have heard of 'food sensitivity tests', which float around on social media, promoted by various different 'health clinics'. These companies ask for a sample of blood, which they expose to various proteins from different foods in test tubes and measure the levels of immunoglobulin G (IgG) antibodies present. The theory goes that the more IgG that shows up in response to a food, the more reactive you are to said food, and that you therefore may be intolerant of it.

This approach is enormously flawed, as when you eat literally anything, your body will trigger an immune response to that food. It's only natural; food is a foreign body entering our gut, so we make immunoglobulins (or antibodies) against that food. The presence of IgG in blood is a marker of tolerance, not intolerance.[9] These IgG tests are also not reliable because they do not measure the severity of the reaction. A person with a high level of antibody to a food may not have symptoms, but someone with low levels of antibodies may have severe symptoms. These IgG tests have never been tested in clinical trials to demonstrate their efficacy. The reason *some* people may benefit from cutting out *some* of these 'triggered' foods (that show up positive on these tests) is simply that they're often high in FODMAPs (which we'll explain later), and the prevalence of IBS is rampant enough for some people to confirm a false observation.

The same can be said about stool microbiome samples (where you send in a bit of poo for analysis, in order to get a snapshot of your microbiome composition). However, that's the entire problem; it's a snapshot of a tiny number of bacteria at an isolated point in time, and as such it should not be used to inform dietary or lifestyle changes. You could argue that with help from a specialized doctor or dietitian, you may be able to trial some dietary changes based on these results with questionable effectiveness, but outside that, they're pretty useless and overstated.

The bottom line: The food sensitivity tests you see advertised online, including IgG blood tests and stool samples, are largely pointless. There are more specific medical tests that can be ordered by your doctor to look for individual intolerances – such as fructose or lactose breath tests – but the most effective way to identify food intolerances is to do an elimination diet and challenge test under the supervision of your medical team.

Microbiome myth no. 4: Artificial sweeteners damage the gut

Artificial or non-nutritive sweeteners (NNS), such as aspartame, sucralose and acesulfame potassium, and their impact on health are one of the most controversial topics in the wellness space today. Ongoing 'incorrect' talks about them causing obesity (covered in the weight-loss chapter), diabetes (via glucose intolerance), heart disease or even cancer remain rife. Yet one of the most heated claims in recent years surrounds their impact on the microbiome, with a handful of studies causing hysteria.

To understand how these sweeteners affect the gut, we first must understand how they're metabolized in the body. Aspartame, for example, is broken down into aspartic acid, phenylalanine and methanol, which is then rapidly absorbed long before it reaches the large bowel, essentially making it unable to harm the microbiota.[10] Whereas other sweeteners such as sucralose or saccharin do reach the large bowel, the research still doesn't indicate anything alarming thus far. Animal studies have suggested that these sweeteners aren't exactly metabolically inert, although we should now be objective enough to realize that the effects found in rodent studies can't be directly translated to humans.

So, what does the human data suggest? The totality of human evidence shows no real concerns.[11] If you're going to make the argument that artificial sweeteners 'harm' or alter the microbiome, then you need to state what the negative effect of that alteration is. Are you suggesting it increases your risk of diabetes? Cancer? What about heart disease? Well, meta-analyses of dozens of controlled and observational human trials show no negative effects on glucose control, body weight, liver health or cancer risk.[12] The fact is, we have forty years' worth of scientific data on these artificial sweeteners, with aspartame being one of the most heavily studied food additives in existence. The scientific consensus from all the major health institutes from around the world remains that artificial sweeteners like aspartame are safe for human consumption with an acceptable daily intake of 40mg/kg. This is the equivalent of a 70kg adult consuming fourteen diet drinks every single day for their entire life.

The bottom line: While it is possible for *some* people to be sensitive to *some* artificial sweeteners, as is the case with almost any food or drink, that does not mean that they damage or 'harm' the gut. Research shows that the common artificial sweeteners are perfectly safe for human consumption and are a great substitute for added sugar.

Best friends in a previous life

Now that we've debunked some of the most common gut-health myths, let's elaborate on the science of the microbiome. Did you know that our encounters with microbes begin even before birth? Even then, the state of our microbiota has in part already been decided for us. It was thought for a long time that the *in utero* (in the womb) environment was a sterile and clean place. However, as a foetus, we consume amniotic fluid that contains an abundance of bacteria – and we even consume our own waste, called meconium.[13]

These free-roaming, *in utero* microbes usually don't get past the oceans of saliva sweeping them away, or survive the harsh environment that waits for them in the stomach's acidic plunge pool. Yet a few lucky explorers will make their way into the intestines and begin designing a new colony there. Further along, the method of delivery also plays a huge impact on the early infant microbiota. During a vaginal birth, the baby's head, eyes, mouth and ears are the first to be colonized as they pass along the mother's soft vaginal wall, where many eager microbes in the moist and warm mucosal layer are waiting to make the leap. Soon after, because of their close proximity and the pressure on the body's sphincters, a light mixture of urinary and faecal microbes are sprinkled onto the baby's face and hands. This is followed by a different set of microbes covering the rest of the baby's body as a result of rubbing against the skin of the mother's legs.

These events lead to a typically stable microbial composition showing an abundance of two species of bacteria: the *Lactobacillus* and *Prevotella* species, which reflects the composition of the vagina.[14] Conversely, babies delivered via caesarean sections are rich in the *Staphylococcus* species, due to its prevalence on the skin as the baby is plucked out of the lower abdomen. There has been some interesting research showing caesarean babies have a higher prevalence of asthma, coeliac disease and type 1 diabetes.[15] This ties in to the 'hygiene hypothesis' that proposes childhood exposure to certain pathogens and infections can help the immune system to develop, thus reducing the risk of allergic and autoimmune diseases.[16] It appears getting squished through the messy, contaminated vaginal wall serves a very real purpose. However, these links between allergic diseases and delivery method are extremely difficult to test, as it's near impossible to isolate the effects of a single exposure from early childhood.

How we were fed as babies also influences our gut composition. Those of us who were breastfed have a higher number of the *Bifidobacterium* bacterial species, which is particularly effective at breaking down human milk sugars, shows anti-inflammatory capabilities and enhances gut barrier function.[17] Whereas infants who were formula-fed have shown higher levels of the pro-inflammatory *Proteobacteria* species. This is why some well-designed interventions have shown that fortifying formula with human milk oligosaccharides (a type of sugar), have shown positive impacts on the microbiome, decreasing risk of infections and inflammatory biomarkers.[18]

These are just some of the reasons why it's arguably better for the child's long-term health to be delivered and fed in natural ways, if possible. As you're reading this, clearly these microbiome-altering events have already been determined for us and there's not much we can change about them now. However, we will dissect the convincing evidence showing that the factors we *can* change, like our diet, play a pivotal role in our microbial make-up and long-term gut health.

The microbiome and obesity

By now you're aware that obesity is not just a simple matter of eating too much and moving too little. It's a complex disease with numerous factors at play. But despite decades of research, we still don't fully understand all the factors that are causing the current epidemic. However, one area of study that's been shedding light on the issue is the gut microbiota – the trillions of microorganisms that live in our digestive tract.

While we've long known that these tiny critters help us break down food and absorb nutrients, recent advances in technology have allowed us to discover far more about their role in weight gain. And what we've discovered is nothing short of fascinating. It turns out that our gut microbiota has a major impact on how much energy we extract from food, as well as on inflammation and the composition of our fat tissue, although it's important to note that the relationship between our gut bacteria and weight gain is not a one-way street. While it's true that shifts in our microbiota can exacerbate the harmful effects of excess weight, the evidence suggests that changes in our diet are actually what drive these shifts in the first place. While some 'gut experts' may be quick to blame our gut bacteria for the obesity epidemic, the truth is much more complex. By continuing to explore the intricate interplay between our microbiota and our bodies, we may one day have the key to tackling this pervasive health issue.

There are apparent differences in the microbial make-up between obese and non-obese people. For example, people with obesity tend to have increased numbers of the bacterial species *Firmicutes* and decreased levels of *Bacteroidetes*.[19] These species-specific differences change when people lose weight, implying that our microbes are constantly changing in response to our body habitus.[20] *Firmicutes* bacteria have been linked to lower resting energy expenditure, whereas low levels of *Bacteroides* are linked to increasing body fat percentages.[21] Interestingly, studies on rodents have shown that transferring a type of the latter, *B. thetaiotaomicron*, to mice that received a normal diet resulted in a significant reduction in total fat and prevented weight gain in rodents that were fed a high-fat diet.[22] Evidence now suggests that the Western dietary pattern is causing alterations in the microbiota, which can increase energy harvesting from food. This is seen in the increase in enzyme activity involved in energy extraction.[23] Simply put, the changes in the gut bacteria caused by the Western diet may lead to you *intaking more calories from the same meal* as someone else with a different dietary pattern – making it exponentially easier to gain weight over time on a Western-style diet.

Another important function of the gut microbiome is the ability to alter bile acid signalling and to produce distinct and unique bile acid profiles.[24] Approximately 5–10 per cent of bile acids are bio-transformed by anaerobic gut microbiota (*Bacteroides*, *Eubacterium* and *Clostridium*), with the rest secreted in our faeces. Variations in bile acid metabolism may increase triglyceride synthesis and lipid (fat) storage in the body.

While these mechanisms are fascinating, it's important to mention that the majority of the aforementioned pathways are derived from animal studies, and there is a lot of inter-individual variability between the composition of the microbiota in lean and obese people. The Human Microbiome Project and Meta-HIT surveyed both lean and obese adults, and found that the composition of stool microbiomes displays large degrees of variability among individuals.[25] So while there are some consistencies with specific microbes in obese versus non-obese adults, a microbial 'signature' of obesity doesn't exist.

Examining this topic with a broader lens, a more accurate conclusion of how the microbiota ties into obesity is that our diet (and the chronic overconsumption of calories) can cause a shift in our gut microbiome, which then enhances the detrimental effects of weight gain, because these bacteria can extract more energy from the same food and increase fat storage in the body. With this in mind, focusing on prebiotic fibres (compounds in food that beneficial bacterial species can feed on and grow) will help to halt these harmful mechanisms. They allow positive bacteria such as *Bifidobacterium* to grow and produce beneficial short-chain fatty acids (SCFAs), as well as reducing the amount of energy we extract from food. Prebiotics are found naturally in garlic, unripe bananas, apples, wheat, barley, soy, oats, onions and leeks.

How the gut impacts cardiometabolic health

As we continue our exploration into the fascinating world of gut health, it's important to take a brief detour and examine the gut–heart–sugar axis. Yes, I just coined that term, but hear me out! While the exact link between our microbiome and cardiometabolic diseases is still being studied, there's no denying the potential impact of our gut on our heart and sugar levels. One way that our gut plays a critical role in our overall health is through its ability to regulate our cholesterol balance.[26] When we consume cholesterol through our diet, our gut is responsible for absorbing it.[27] But here's where things get interesting: our microbiome can actually influence the composition of our blood lipids, which can have a direct impact on the development of coronary artery disease. For example, certain types of gut bacteria, like *Lactobacillus reuteri*, have been linked to higher levels of ('good') HDL cholesterol, while others, like *Eggerthella*, have been linked to lower levels.[28] But that's not all. Chronic inflammation in the gut has also been linked to atherosclerosis, a process in which immune cells trigger inflammation in the arteries. However, research has shown that certain inflammatory cytokines, like interleukin-22, can help protect the gut lining and reduce inflammation throughout the body.

One nutrient that reduces cardiovascular and metabolic disease via mechanisms in the gut is soluble fibre. Increasing fibres with greater solubility and viscosity from foods like oats, peas, beans, apples and citrus fruits has been shown to delay gastric emptying, slowing down digestion and coating the lining of the gut – which decreases the absorption of macronutrients. The properties of these fibres result in a lower postprandial (after a meal) blood glucose and insulin level.[29] Furthermore, fibre promotes the production of growth hormones and the growth of beneficial bacteria that produce SCFAs, which have various metabolic benefits for the heart and liver. Fibre also plays a key role in managing total calorie intake and has the highest thermic effect of food after protein.[30] It's because of mechanisms like these that new meta-analyses of hundreds of observational and controlled studies show that fibre intake reduces your blood pressure, fasting glucose and LDL cholesterol, all of which are key layers in the development of cardiometabolic diseases.[31] This further strengthens the advice to consume a variety of different fibre types on a daily basis.

The gut–brain axis

As medicine advances and becomes more specialized, I can't help but think how we are losing track of the big picture, focusing on single organs to determine what is wrong with someone, to then treat them based on that specific organ. It's a fundamental flaw in the healthcare system, whereby the burden is put on the primary-care physician to identify the links between bodily systems. Granted, we've come a long way from the cold showers and shackles of the eighteenth century; 200 years ago, 'madness' was considered an evil state and the mentally ill were locked in prisons. The issue is, we've become more and more focused on the emotions and thought processes of mental illness (which is a good thing), and stopped noticing that the rest of the body is also involved.

Historian Ian Miller reminds us that the nineteenth-century medical community acknowledged a profound link between our stomachs and minds, a notion they termed 'nervous sympathy'.[32] Fast-forward to today, and research on the gut–brain axis has surged, revealing the interconnectedness of our gut, central nervous system and behaviour – largely steered by our microbiome's impact on our emotional health. What was once perceived as a startling revelation – the impact of gut health on emotional well-being – has now become widely accepted, marking a paradigm shift in medicine. The advent of 'psychobiotics' – beneficial bacteria acting on the gut–brain axis, sometimes with antidepressant effects – underscores this new perspective. Today's Western world, plagued by the twin epidemics of mental health and gut issues, can no longer ignore their interplay. In this section, we will delve into the complexities of the gut–brain axis and its implications for our health.

When you consider the gut's mysterious ability to communicate with the brain, it's really illogical to conclude that it doesn't play a vital role in our state of mind. A plethora of recent studies indicate that the gut microbiome's importance goes beyond our physical health. It's also a key player in the gut–brain connection. Thirty-something years ago, a very influential trial was conducted which showed for the first time that changing our gut's bacterial composition could alter our mental function.[33] Researchers tested this on a series of patients with hepatic encephalopathy (a severe form of liver disease that causes a build-up of toxins in the blood and brain, resulting in delirium and confusion). The main toxin of concern here is ammonia, which is produced by harmful bacteria. The patients were administered with a specific type of oral antibiotics, which lowered blood toxin levels and improved delirium by decreasing the number of ammonia-producing bacteria in the colon. These findings were huge. The hypothesis that changing our gut bacteria can improve our mental function has also been demonstrated multiple times in rodent trials, where a strain of timid mice was given a cocktail of antibiotics that completely changed their behaviour, making them adventurous and bold.[34]

While most research on the gut–brain axis in humans is still in its early stages, there is some evidence of the microbiome's potential to impact stress, anxiety, depression and even neurological conditions like autism spectrum disorder. A study conducted in

2011 found that probiotics significantly reduced psychological distress by improving anxiety, depression, stress and cortisol scores.[35] This was possibly due to certain gut bacteria introduced by the probiotics, which produced short-chain fatty acids crucial for inflammation reduction and brain health. There's also exciting research suggesting that gut-produced SCFAs can increase the production of brain-derived neurotrophic factor (BDNF), an essential protein for memory and mood, and help to mitigate neuroinflammation.[36]

Disruptions in the gut microbiome, known as gut dysbiosis, can influence the metabolism of tryptophan, an amino acid precursor to serotonin. High activity of the enzyme indoleamine oxidase (IDO), which is responsible for metabolizing tryptophan, can lead to decreased serotonin production. This pathway has been implicated in disorders like IBS and depression.[37] Research also indicates a link between altered gut bacteria and conditions such as autism and Parkinson's disease, with higher levels of harmful bacteria correlating with more severe symptoms.[38]

Most research into the gut–brain axis is now only in its preliminary stages, but one intervention that has proven to be effective in modulating stress is the consumption of fermented milk topped with probiotics. A couple of studies have found drinks like this cause changes on functional magnetic resonance imaging (fMRI) scanning that improved the ability to process emotions.[39] This doesn't mean we all should start taking probiotics right away; as we saw earlier, it's a little more complicated than that. The strongest evidence to date suggests that changing gut bacteria can improve anxiety, stress, depression and improve symptoms of various brain disorders by increasing SFCA-producing bacteria to then reduce neuroinflammation. The point is, anyone making confident claims or prescriptive recommendations regarding how the gut microbiome is linked to mental health is largely talking rubbish.

Inflammatory bowel disease

Inflammatory bowel disease (IBD) is a common, chronic, immune-mediated disease affecting the gastrointestinal tract. In the United States, it is estimated that over 3 million adults (1.3 per cent of the population) have been diagnosed with IBD as of 2015. IBD consists of two subtypes: ulcerative colitis and Crohn's disease. It's not exactly clear why IBD arises, but genetics, environmental factors and having an altered microbiota all play a role.

There are several mechanisms by which a typical Western diet can increase the risk of IBD and colorectal cancer. The consumption of an animal-based, high-saturated-fat and no-fibre diet has been shown in controlled human trials to rapidly shift microbial composition.[40] In one study, researchers prepared two diets: a plant-based diet rich in grains, legumes, fruits and vegetables; and an animal-based diet comprising meats, eggs and cheese. They saw that the animal-based diet increased the numbers of bile-tolerant organisms (*Bilophila* and *Bacteroides*) and decreased levels of helpful *Firmicutes*. Enhanced activity of *Bilophila* microbes can lead to pro-inflammatory bacterial species, along with nitrogenous metabolites – together, these can induce intestinal inflammation and the growth of cancerous cells.[41]

Here are two key nutrients that can improve the composition of the gut microbiota and help those with IBD:

- **Omega-3** fatty acids may improve quality of life for people with IBD by helping to stabilize the disease. Studies have found that mice – which are prone to gut inflammation (colitis) and consuming a high-fat diet – saw a reduction in the growth of harmful bacteria *B. wadsworthia* when fed fish oils. This led to a reduced likelihood of developing colitis.[42] The most comprehensive meta-analysis of eighty-three RCTs in humans, looking specifically at polyunsaturated fats on inflammatory bowel disease, found that omega-3s may reduce the risk of IBD relapse and worsening of symptoms, yet didn't significantly alter systemic inflammatory markers.[43]

- **Vitamin D** is perhaps of greater interest, as trials in patients with Crohn's disease show that each 1ng/mL increase in plasma vitamin D levels leads to a 8 per cent reduction in the risk of colorectal cancer.[44] Supplementing with 1200IU/d of vitamin D3 for a year reduced the risk of relapse from 29 per cent to 13 per cent, and a high dose of 10,000IU/d appears to reduce the rate of relapse even further.[45] These effects are seen due to vitamin D's ability to increase antimicrobial activity (e.g. facilitating macrophages in killing *E. coli*), maintain the integrity of the intestinal lining and prevent harmful shifts in bacterial species, which in turn inhibits inflammatory processes.[46] Depending on baseline levels, supplementing with 2,000–10,000IU/d of vitamin D to achieve a plasma level of >50ng/mL appears to be beneficial in managing IBD and improving gut functionality. But what should you do if you experience a flare-up of IBD?

When I was working regularly on general surgical wards, IBD flare-ups were a daily sight. I remember a young patient, Alexis, with ulcerative colitis. Feverish, doubled over in pain, his frustration was palpable. He had suffered multiple flare-ups within a short period of time and was adamant that he wanted a surgery called a proctocolectomy – which involves removal of the colon and rectum – despite the temporary ostomy bag that would become a permanent part of his life.

His issue was his diet. During flare-ups, he would temporarily cut out fibrous foods, spices and more robust flavours, which helped to ease his pain. Once he felt better, he would straight away revert back to a fibre-rich diet, leading to more pain and another flare-up. This cycle raised an important question: why would high fibre – a commonly accepted gut-booster – exacerbate his condition?

The answer lies in the complexity of the microbiome. While sudden high-fibre intakes can worsen symptoms in disrupted microbiomes and IBD, long-term high-fibre diets actually reduce IBD relapse rates and risk.[47] An analysis of eight studies even revealed a 13 per cent reduction in Crohn's disease risk with every 10g increase in daily fibre.[48] A different study compared high-fibre and fermented-food diets over ten weeks.[49] Interestingly, the fermented-food diet group showed reductions in inflammatory proteins, increased gut microbial diversity, and decreased immune cell activity. Meanwhile, some on the high-fibre diet experienced increased inflammation, suggesting that loading up an unprepared gut with lots of fibre may not be beneficial. A gradual increase in fibre, perhaps coupled with fermented foods that add fibre-consuming microbes, may be more advantageous. Although avoiding fibre provides temporary relief during IBD flare-ups and those suffering with gut issues, it shouldn't be mistaken as a long-term solution. While claims of healing gut issues with an animal-based diet are widespread, they often overlook the resulting decline in microbial diversity and long-term health.

Ensuring adequate omega-3 intakes, exposure to sunlight and dietary and supplemental intakes of vitamin D can all help manage relapses and intestinal health in IBD. After a flare-up of IBD, when you'd likely want to eliminate fibre and spice intake for a while, look to slowly reintroduce fibrous foods. Over several weeks, perhaps include a single serving of fruits, grains, vegetables or legumes daily, and slowly increase your fibre intake every few days. Giving your body time to adjust to these fibrous foods can allow beneficial bacterial species to grow in sufficient quantities, which can then adequately break down these fibres and produce healthful metabolites for your gut and body. This will reduce the risk of another flare-up, allow your body to handle all kinds of foods, improve symptoms and benefit overall metabolic health by ensuring a rich and diverse microbiome.

Now, let's tackle IBS in more detail and explore the most effective strategies we have to help combat it.

Irritable bowel syndrome

IBS is an extremely common condition that describes a group of symptoms: bloating, abdominal pain, diarrhoea or constipation (or both). It's estimated to affect between 9 and 23 per cent of the population across the entire world.[50] The cause of IBS is not clear, but historically it's been recognized for over 150 years. In 1849, the scientist William Cumming reported 'the bowels are at one time constipated, another lax, in the same person. How the disease has two such different symptoms I do not profess to explain.'[51]

Many things can lead to IBS, such as subtle intestinal inflammation, altered motility of the bowel, post-infectious reactivity, gut–brain interactions through stress or anxiety manifestations, food sensitivities and bacterial overgrowth.[52] Have you ever been extremely nervous about something, perhaps an interview, a date or a sports competition, and just had raging diarrhoea out of nowhere? Exactly . . . That's the power of the gut–brain axis.

The treatment of IBS is multifaceted, requiring a tailored history and examination, dietary advice and medication to help different types of IBS, as well as stress or anxiety management. Typical dietary advice includes promoting balanced nutrient profiles while reducing fatty food, alcohol, stimulants like caffeine, and going easy on the spice.

One nutritional strategy has been effective in more than 75 per cent of IBS sufferers: the low-FODMAP diet. FODMAP stands for 'fermentable oligo-, di- and monosaccharides and polyols' – which are all specific types of carbohydrates. Many people with digestive symptoms find these carbs seem to trigger their symptoms, because they draw more fluid into the intestine. Due to their nature, they are more easily fermented in the gut, and the combination of fluid and gas can slow digestion, resulting in pain, bloating or diarrhoea. This is why a meta-analysis of twelve controlled trials showed that following a low-FODMAP diet significantly reduced gastrointestinal symptoms and improved quality of life.[53]

Currently, advisory bodies like the American College of Gastroenterology and the British Dietetic Association advise that a low-FODMAP diet should be implemented as a first- and second-line treatment for IBS.[54] It's sometimes a long process of trial and error to pinpoint precisely which foods are the triggers. It may seem daunting at first, but the aim isn't to restrict all these foods, it's to find those that trigger you, cut them out and work on reintroducing them back into your diet over time. Finding the foods that trigger your symptoms typically follows a three-step process:

1. **Elimination** – eliminate all FODMAP carbs for several weeks. Your symptoms may improve immediately or over several weeks. If symptoms are successfully reduced within 6–8 weeks then you can move on to step 2.
2. **Reintroduction** – introduce one FODMAP at a time to identify which foods you can tolerate and in what quantities.
3. **Personalization** – you'll want to modify your diet to increase variety while adjusting the type and amount of FODMAP carbs you eat, based on what you learned in step 2.

HIGH-FODMAP CARBS YOU SHOULD INITIALLY AVOID

- **Fructose** – fruits (specifically apples, mangoes, pears, watermelon), honey, high fructose corn syrup, agave

- **Lactose** – dairy (milk from cows, goats or sheep), custard, yoghurt, ice cream
- **Fructans** – rye and wheat, asparagus, broccoli, cabbage, onions, garlic
- **Galactans** – legumes such as beans, lentils, chickpeas and soybeans
- **Polyols** – sugar alcohols and fruits with pits or seeds (apples, apricots, avocados, cherries, figs, peaches, pears and plums)

These can be reintroduced one by one as per step 2.

LOW-FODMAP FOODS TO ENJOY INSTEAD

- **Fruit** – bananas, blueberries, grapefruit, kiwi, lemon, lime, oranges, strawberries
- **Dairy** – almond milk, lactose-free milk, coconut milk, lactose-free yoghurt and hard cheeses (e.g. mature cheddar or parmesan)
- **Vegetables** – beansprouts, carrots, chives, cucumber, ginger, lettuce, potatoes, parsnips, turnips, spring onion, bok choy
- **Protein** – beef, pork, chicken, fish, eggs, tofu
- **Nuts/seeds** – (limit to 15 each) almonds, peanuts, pine nuts and walnuts
- **Grains** – oats, oat bran, gluten-free pasta, white rice, quinoa, corn flour and rice bran

In addition to specific carbs, positive associations exist between fat intake and an increase in stool number and diarrhoea. On the other hand, soluble fibre results in an improvement in IBS symptomology and constipation.[55]

In summary, effective treatment of IBS requires attention to all aspects of your lifestyle: stress and anxiety management, identification of food intolerances and triggers, regular exercise habits and working to build a healthy gut microbiome. A good way in which to start is restricting high-FODMAP foods, and prioritizing a low-FODMAP diet with the aim of identifying triggers and reintroducing foods over time.

Fibre and the microbiome

As fibre is a major component of optimizing gut health, I want to briefly characterize what fibre actually is, and summarize its main role of the microbiome and why it's important for our health. Fibre is a type of carbohydrate that the body cannot break down, so it passes through our gut into our large intestine. It is found naturally in plant foods like whole grains, beans, nuts, seeds, fruits and veg, and is sometimes added to foods and drink. 'Fibre' is an umbrella term for hundreds of different types of fibre, and each fibre has differing proportions of three main characteristics:

1. **Solubility** – it draws water into the gut, softens stools and regulates metabolic health
2. **Viscosity** – it swells food to form a thick jelly-like mass, slows digestion, aids satiety and has metabolic benefits
3. **Fermentability** – it has the ability to feed and grow healthy bacteria

It's important to be aware that not all fibre is the same. For example, while psyllium husk (from the *Plantago ovata* seed husk) and inulin (found in garlic, agave, bananas and onions) are both 'soluble fibre', they look extremely different and have different functions. Psyllium is granular, makes a thick gel and is inaccessible to fibre-degrading bacteria, but it does help with bowel function. Inulin, on the other hand, is dissolved in water, has no thickness and acts as a fertilizer to the gut bacteria, making it a prebiotic. As such, the old-school classification of soluble versus insoluble doesn't adequately categorize fibre in any meaningful way.

This level of nuance becomes important when dealing with certain medical conditions. Psyllium husk is particularly effective at treating constipation (as it acts as a bulking agent to facilitate healthy bowel movements),[56] whereas inulin could make constipation worse (because of the fermentation process in the gut).[57] When our microbes feed on inulin, gas is released and acidic by-products which act on our enteric nervous system (the nervous system of the gastrointestinal tract) can cause discomfort, bloating and pain. For most people, simply advising that they aim to regularly consume a variety of plant fibres weekly should be enough, although we must be aware that certain medical conditions and symptoms will require an individualized approach.

Intermittent fasting and microbes

Many environmental and genetic factors play a role in influencing the gut microbiota, but one field of research that is gaining tremendous traction is the topic of intermittent or periodic fasting. Intermittent fasting has been shown to provide favourable effects on obesity, metabolic, cardiovascular and neurodegenerative diseases, yet recent evidence suggests the effects of fasting and feeding patterns on metabolism can be closely linked with alterations in our gut bacterial species.

A recent systematic review of thirty-one studies on both animals and humans found that intermittent fasting (including Ramadan) enhanced beneficial bacterial species including *Lactobacillus* and *Bifidobacterium*.[58] Several mechanisms are said to be responsible for these positive adaptations. Changes in the gut microbiome from fasting have been shown to increase energy expenditure by converting white adipose tissue to brown adipose tissue, which appears to be more metabolically active.[59] Intermittent fasting also allows sufficient time for microbial fermentation to take place in the gut, which in turn increases positive by-products including the previously mentioned SCFAs. We've established that losing weight positively impacts bacterial species, and intermittent fasting is a method to achieve calorie restriction, which also benefits systemic and gut-specific inflammation although it's difficult to tease out what percentage of the benefits are due to calorie restriction or whether inherent benefits exist from the fasting itself.

The guts of the matter

Scientific research on how the gut microbiome impacts health is still in its infancy. The gut is vastly complicated, and due to huge inter-individual variability (we have literally trillions of microbes within each of us), it's difficult to give blanket recommendations across the board. That being said, at the broadest level we do have some key nutritional principles that are proven to increase the bacterial species associated with positive health outcomes.

Key takeaways

1. **Branch out.** The more diverse an array of plant-based foods you consume, the more diverse your bacterial growth (crucial for adequate metabolic balancing) will be. Fibre plays a key role in shaping the microbiome and reducing the risk of cardiometabolic diseases such as heart disease, fatty liver and type 2 diabetes. Evidence suggests that the optimal diet to support the gut includes a proportion of fibre well above the levels found in the

typical Western diet, and research from the American Gut Project shows that those who consume thirty different plants per week have a more diverse microbiome compared to those who eat ten per week.[60] Aim for 30–50g of fibre per day from 20–30 different plant-based foods per week. 30g of fibre looks something like this:

- 5 servings of veg
- 2 servings of fruit
- 3 servings of whole grains
- 3 servings of legumes, nuts or seeds

2. **No no, not for you!** The beauty of prebiotic fibres is that they are resistant to stomach acid, enzymes and absorption in the small intestine, enabling them to make their way to the large intestine and provide food for our little best friends. This results in the growth and activity of our microbes, in turn improving our mental health, gastrointestinal lining, cardiometabolic health and energy processing. Make sure to regularly include fibre-rich foods like oats, barley, wheat, soybeans, garlic, unripe bananas, apples, onions, asparagus and leeks.

3. **Put down the steak.** A diet that is high in animal fats and animals appears to be harmful to the composition and normal functioning of the gut microbiota, based on the strongest evidence. Saturated fats are known to increase the production of bile acid, thus enhancing acid-tolerant bacteria, whereas unsaturated fats prevent the growth of these harmful bacterial groups by altering the structure of bile acid. Aim to reduce fatty cuts of red meat and replace them with fatty fish, skinless chicken, turkey breast and plant proteins such as soy, peas, tempeh and legumes.

4. **Omega-3 and vitamin D play an important role** in our gut wall integrity, inhibiting harmful microbial activity and maintaining remission in IBD. Try to eat a couple of servings of salmon, mackerel, soybeans, flaxseeds and chia seeds per week, and if possible allow the sun to hit your skin for about twenty minutes a day.

5. **Be careful with elimination diets.** Cutting out plant-based foods through an elimination or low-FODMAP diet does play a role in managing many conditions such as IBS, intolerances and IBD. However, this should be a temporary measure only. When your symptoms have resolved, the microbiome is no longer equipped to deal with beneficial plant-based foods, which is why consuming them can make you feel unpleasant. Instead of avoiding plant-based foods for good, aim to slowly reintroduce them over a period of weeks, with the intention of increasing the dosage and frequency gradually to allow the body time to adapt.

6. **Eat fermented foods rather than taking probiotic supplements.** Despite having some therapeutic benefits in specific disease states, investing in probiotic supplements will likely be a waste of money. You're much better off ditching the supplements and focusing on fermented foods such as fermented yoghurts and milk, kombucha, kefir, sauerkraut, pickles, sourdough bread and cheese.

7. **The gut–everything axis!** Every single food we eat will have an effect on our microbiome, whether it's positive or negative. Our gut health is closely linked to all the chapters we discuss in this book. It's important to acknowledge that these topics are not mutually exclusive – they all fit together and play a crucial role in preventing and managing chronic lifestyle disease.

Depression and Dementia

Feeding Your Feelings

In the previous chapter we uncovered the critical role the micro-biome plays in digestion, immunity and even regulating our mood. We unveiled the intricate interactions within this internal ecosystem, painting a picture of an unseen world with profound impacts on our health and well-being. In this new chapter we will explore the connection between our diet and the brain, starting with an area of mental health of urgent concern – depression – followed by the leading cause of death in the UK: dementia.

Depression, a common and debilitating mental health disorder, continues to impact millions of lives worldwide, with its origins and treatment often proving elusive. Despite advancements in medical science, the comprehensive understanding and management of depression remain a challenge. An emerging area of research, however, offers promising insight into the pivotal role of nutrition and the gut–brain axis in influencing our mood and mental health. Our diet not only provides us with the energy we need to function physically, it also plays a crucial role in determining the diversity and function of our gut microbiota, which subsequently impact our mental health.

Drawing on the most recent scientific studies, in this chapter we will unravel how our daily dietary choices can influence our mood and mental health via the gut–brain axis, a bidirectional communication pathway linking the central nervous system with the gastrointestinal tract. We will also explore how adopting a balanced, nutrient-rich diet can help us offer potential preventative measures and treatment strategies for depression.

Diet and depression

I still remember my first day working as part of the psychiatry liaison team like it was yesterday. I was feeling a mixture of nervousness and excitement. I had just been given the instruction from my consultant: 'Dr Mughal, there's a patient on ward 14 that is due for a Mental Health Act assessment in an hour, go with Dr Asif to meet the external psychiatrist and social worker and assist them.' The MHA assessment is one of the most critical tools in all of psychiatry. It's a decision that can alter the course of a patient's life forever. The assessment determines whether a patient needs to be detained in a hospital against their will in order to receive treatment for their underlying mental health condition.

This particular patient was an eighteen-year-old with emotionally unstable personality disorder (EUPD), who had experienced a horrific upbringing. I had dealt with all kinds of poorly and complex patients before, but there was something about mental health illness that kept me on edge. Perhaps it was the stigmatization of mental health by other medical specialities. Or the notion that psychiatry doctors are somehow lesser, because you cannot see what it is they're treating. There are no blood tests, no X-rays to identify the problem, just a room full of 'crazies', as I'd heard even my colleagues say sometimes. Or perhaps it was the depictions of mentally ill people in countless psychological thrillers on Netflix. Whatever it was, I knew that I needed to keep my composure and approach the situation with professionalism and empathy.

As I entered the ward with Dr Asif, I felt a sense of unease wash over me. We were about to make a decision that would change the life of a young woman forever. The gravity of the situation was palpable. The young woman in question had been in and out of social and psychiatric care so many times that she

new exactly what it meant to see multiple doctors. Her resist-
nce was expected, but her reaction was something I had never
een before. As soon as we entered the room, she started thrash-
ng and screaming, swinging her limbs around in every direction.
: was as if she had become a completely different person, and I
vas speechless. I couldn't help but wonder how she had come to
e in such a state.

In situations like this, it is compulsory to have at least two doc-
ors and an approved mental health professional present. We
eeded to make sure that every possible option was explored
efore we made any major decisions. Unfortunately, as is often
he case, we had to resort to restraining, sedating and sectioning
er, until she could be transferred to a mental health hospital. It
vas a difficult decision to make, but we knew that it was the best
hing for her in the long run. As we left the ward, I felt sad. It was
lear that this young woman needed intensive psychological ther-
py and it was up to us to make sure that she received the help
hat she needed.

When you think about mental health treatment, you might
icture a therapist's couch or a box of pills as possible solutions.
ut while conditions such as EUPD are clearly caused by com-
lex factors, and dietary changes alone won't make much of an
npact, we do now know that diet can play a key role in manag-
ng symptoms and improving quality of life for those suffering
rith various other mental health disorders. Nutrition and mental
ealth may not seem like the most obvious partners, but the field
f nutritional psychiatry is one that is growing exponentially.

Medical professionals are only now starting to understand the
ple that diet plays in our mental health. The brain is always
ctive. It looks after our thoughts, movements, breath, heartbeat
nd almost every other bodily function you can think of. It is con-
antly working, even while we're asleep. This requires a large
mount of energy on a daily basis, and that energy comes from
ood. It is only logical to suggest that the types of food we choose

to consume will affect our brain's ability to perform and keep u:
healthy.

It is no coincidence that the change in our food environmen
over the last few decades is being reflected in the current menta
health state of the West. One in five American adults will have ;
diagnosable mental health condition in any given year, while ar
astonishing 46 per cent will meet the criteria for a mental healtl
condition at some point in their lives. Meanwhile, depression i:
set to become the leading cause of disability by the year 2030 ir
high-income countries,[1] something which we'll dive into shortly
We have become infatuated with the power of wonder drugs anc
the supplement market as a one-stop resolution strategy. The sac
reality is, drugs can only do so much – and in the case of demen
tia, which we'll tackle later, most pharmaceuticals that are
developed and tested don't even make it to market.

Diet and mood fact no. 1: Food significantly affects your mood

Depression affects more than 264 million people around the
world and leads about 800,000 people to commit suicide every
year.[2] It is the fourth leading cause of death in 15- to 29-year-olds
It is common in every country of the world, with the United
States coming out on top and China and Japan being the leas
affected. It is a leading cause of disability globally,[3] and entails tre
mendous suffering and loss of functionality – which can impai
performance at work and school and strain relationships witl
loved ones.

This was evident to me when I was working as a psychiatry
doctor. One day I met a young 42-year-old gentleman (young b}
hospital standards, at least) called Matthew. He was in betweer
jobs, unhappy with his weight, stressed about his family relation
ships and using food to cope and feel better. While he was stil

generally able to function, it was clear he was feeling very low. He had been living by himself and suffering with depression for several years by the time I met him. His evenings were the same every single day: he would come home from work, eat a microwave meal from his local Tesco, sit down to watch TV, open his snack cupboard and freezer and start nibbling on ice cream and chocolate fingers, all the while enjoying a couple of beers. We started exploring his symptoms, and soon something became abundantly clear. Matthew's only outlet for his sadness was food.

I'm sure you know as well as I do how tempting it is to drown any sorrows in alcohol, ice cream and biscuits. Who doesn't love a good mint-chocolate-chip scoop? Even though I'm a doctor and 'should know better', I'm also human and have on many occasions given in to the temptation of 'feeding my feelings'. When stress is creeping up and your mood is plunging, when irritability peaks and your patience is non-existent – it's only natural to turn to comfort food.

But here's the interesting thing. Even though these comfort foods may make us feel better in the short term, the long-term consequences represent a vicious cycle, both physically and mentally. The physical damage of Matthew's comfort- or stress-eating was clear; he gained around 25kg in a short period of time and became diabetic. But the mental toll was even more profound. While Matthew thought that his eating habits were combating his depression, they were actually deepening it.

How often do you, like Matthew, find yourself in a slump, in front of the TV, with a tub of ice cream or a tube of Pringles in hand? A cross-sectional study of university students found that in the 18 per cent of men and 28 per cent of women who had symptoms of depression, 30 per cent ate fried foods, 49 per cent consumed sugary drinks and 52 per cent ate sugary foods more than once per week.[4] In women, a higher depression score was associated with a twofold increased frequency of fast food and fried and sugary foods, suggesting that women are even more susceptible to unhealthy dietary choices when depressed. It goes without saying that not everyone who is depressed binge-eats 'junk food', because depression is extremely complex and can affect appetite and food choices differently. Some people stop eating altogether and experience a markedly reduced appetite,[5] while others become human food-compost bins.

Depression is tied to waning levels of mood-regulating neurotransmitters such as serotonin, changes in brain activity in the mesocorticolimbic reward pathway (the collection of connected brain areas that play a key role in feeling pleasure, motivation and reward) and hypoactivation of insular regions (parts of the brain that help process emotions, the awareness of one's bodily sensations and the feeling of certain tastes).[6] These changes can make normal self-care like cooking a balanced meal extremely challenging. Anhedonia, a very common symptom in clinical depression, is the loss of pleasure in things you usually like to do, which can often relate to food habits. The thought of food and the act of eating, and even preparing food, should be pleasurable and not feel like a burden. Instead, many people with depression want to 'feel better', but convenience food is the easiest option in that moment.

The bottom line: Food drastically affects our mental health, and not enough emphasis is placed on the role that nutrition plays in depression. A single meal can significantly affect how you feel, and a person's total dietary pattern can significantly impact their risk of depression.*[7]

---

* Before diving into the research surrounding diet and depression, it's important to highlight some differences between the sexes. A meta-analysis of sixteen RCTs found that studies using primarily female samples observed significant mental health benefits from dietary interventions, whereas those with male samples did not. Gender differences could potentially be explained by three sex-specific factors. First, women have a higher presence of mood disorders across the population, which may allow for a greater benefit in mood from dietary changes. Second, differences in dietary effects could be linked to sex differences in

Diet and mood fact no. 2: That sweet treat you use as a pick-me-up may be putting you down

Who doesn't love a chocolate bar or a delicious slice of cake when they're feeling low? Refined sugar often feels like a remedy for boredom, anxiety or stress. Refined sugars are those that have been extracted from a natural source – usually from sugar cane, dairy or fruits – and then added to a food product. Now, although refined sugars are chemically identical to the fructose found in fruit, the sucrose found in sugar cane and the lactose found in dairy, there is one fundamental difference. They are no longer in the natural form they once were. The issue with this is that they have been stripped of the fibre, phytochemicals, protein (from dairy), vitamins and minerals that are health-promoting. This is why you hear many people say 'well, natural sugars are good for you, but processed sugars are bad'.

When looking at refined sugars in the context of mental health, there are several plausible biological mechanisms for why they might increase the risk of depression. Firstly, as we discovered in the inflammation chapter, refined sugars are high on the DII and are pro-inflammatory by definition when consumed in large quantities. This increases levels of neuroinflammation and damages the connections in the brain responsible for regulating mood. Secondly, the hippocampus (a small region in the brain that plays a crucial role in the formation of new memories, spatial navigation and emotional regulation) can be affected by sugar intake.

---

metabolism and body composition – women may be more responsive to diets that alter glucose or fat metabolism. Lastly, sociocultural differences between men and women exist regarding diet and health beliefs. Evidence shows that men generally rate health behaviours like diet as being less important than women do; men also have lower nutrition knowledge and women seek nutrition counselling or advice more frequently than men. Therefore, women may be more likely to adopt and benefit from recommended dietary and health behaviours.

Higher sugar intakes are linked to hippocampal wasting or atrophy,[8] and the hippocampus can be up to 25 per cent smaller in depressed people.

Part of the reason this occurs is because of sugar's effect on the protein brain-derived neurotrophic factor (BDNF). The BDNF gene is crucial for the survival of neurons, growth and maturation of nerve cells. A higher-sugar diet has been shown to suppress the production of BDNF, which in turn damages the hippocampus, making us less able to regulate our mood. Converging lines of evidence implicate BDNF in the pathophysiology of major depression. A meta-analysis of eleven studies found a strong connection between lower levels of BDNF and worsening mental health. Interestingly, after treatment with antidepressant medication, participants' BDNF levels increased, suggesting that lower levels of BDNF play a causal role in the initiation of depression.[9]

High glycaemic-index or GI diets (diets rich in refined sugars, lacking healthy fats and fibre) can cause a drastic spike in insulin levels, sometimes leading to temporary hypoglycaemia (a drop below normal blood sugar levels) a few hours after a meal. This can even happen in those without insulin resistance or diabetes and is called reactive hypoglycaemia.[10] It is estimated that up to 50 per cent of US adults are insulin-resistant, so the chances are this is happening more often than people realize.[11] Fluctuating blood sugar levels are linked to cognitive decline (which we'll cover in the dementia section) as well as fluctuating mood states, thus increasing the risk of depression.[12] A recent meta-analysis of ten observational studies and 365,000 participants on sugar-sweetened beverages (SSBs) found that they increase the risk of depression.[13] SSBs are notoriously bad for spiking blood sugar levels, as they contain nothing but sugar and water and therefore have a high glycaemic load. The researchers found that two cups of sugary drink per day were enough to significantly increase depression risk, with the highest sugary drink group having a 31 per cent increased risk compared to the lowest-intake group. An additional proposed mechanism behind these findings is that sugar intake alters endorphin levels and oxidative stress, leading to a greater risk of depression.

In response, people might argue, 'Could it not just be the depression leading people to eat more sugary foods, and not the sugar causing depression itself?' Good question! In research, we call this the 'reverse causation' hypothesis, whereby if you want to know which came first – the chicken or the egg – then you need to have measured people's mood and eating habits at multiple time points to understand the causation sequence. Luckily for us, studies have tested this exact question. The Whitehall II study on over 10,000 British civil servants assessed people's moods and diets every other year for over a decade.[14] They found that people consuming the greatest number of added sugars had a 23 per cent increased risk of depressive symptoms over five years – and the sugar-rich diet tended to precede the onset of depressive symptoms. Not to mention my own research study (which I hope to publish soon) in which I analysed data from over 15,000 twins in the TwinsUK cohort. I found that for every 100g of total sugar intake, there was a 34–41 per cent increased risk of depression – this association held in the longitudinal (over time) analysis too.

The bottom line: Though the occasional refined-sugar treat is obviously not a concern, focusing on natural sugars from fruits and dairy – while reducing our 'added sugar' intake from ultra-processed foods like sweets, biscuits, cakes and ready meals – is an essential part of improving our mental health.

Diet and mood fact no. 3: Artificial sweeteners likely don't impact mood

While reducing refined-sugar intake can improve depressive symptoms, substituting it with zero-calorie alternatives like aspartame, which is found in diet soft drinks, has raised concerns among some. Studies show that high doses of aspartame can lead to negative neurobehavioural side effects such as irritability, depression and poor spatial orientation.[15] However, the doses used in these studies are significantly higher than what an average adult consumes (as high as ten cans of diet cola every day!). Compare this to studies on women who were given standard doses of aspartame over four weeks and found no differences in their mood.[16]

The bottom line: While there are documented side effects, using artificial sweeteners as a substitute for sugar can still benefit mental health. But if you suffer from depression and consume very high amounts of artificially sweetened drinks, reducing or eliminating them may help.

Dietary advice for depression

Now that we've highlighted how certain foods can increase your risk of depression, it's time to learn more about how diet can aid our mental health. Excitingly, each of the following dietary approaches has been shown to decrease depressive symptoms in a recent systematic review of multiple studies, with one study (on the ModiMedDiet) revealing a substantial positive impact.[17]

The ModiMedDiet

This is a modified version of the well-known Mediterranean diet. It revolves around twelve key food groups, as follows:

- whole grains (5–8 servings per day)
- vegetables (6 per day)
- fruit (3 per day), legumes (3–4 per week)
- low-fat and unsweetened dairy foods (2–3 per day)
- raw and unsalted nuts (1 per day)
- fish rich in omega-3 (at least 2 per week)
- lean red meats (3–4 per week)
- chicken (2–3 per week)
- eggs (up to 6 per week)
- olive oil (3 tbsp per day)

While the intake of 'extra' foods (as follows) is reduced or cut completely:

- sweets
- refined cereals
- fried food
- fast food
- processed meats
- sugary drinks (no more than 3 per week)
- alcohol

The ModiMedDiet shares many similarities to the traditional Mediterranean diet, with a few key differences:

- **Red and processed meats:** The ModiMedDiet explicitly advises limiting red meat and completely avoiding processed meats, which might not be as explicitly emphasized in some descriptions of the Mediterranean diet.
- **Recommendation on sweets:** The ModiMedDiet particularly emphasizes a reduction in sweets, refined cereals, fried foods, fast foods and sugary drinks.
- **Alcohol:** While moderate wine consumption, particularly red wine, is a component of the traditional Mediterranean diet (especially when consumed with meals), the ModiMedDiet advises limiting alcoholic

beverages. This is especially relevant given the link between excessive alcohol consumption and depression.

- **Dairy:** The traditional Mediterranean diet often includes yoghurt and cheese, while the ModiMedDiet might have a reduced focus on dairy and emphasizes low-fat varieties.

In one study based around the ModiMedDiet, an impressive 30 per cent of participants saw such significant improvement in their depressive symptoms that they were classified as 'in remission'.[18] This incredible result suggests that even in severe or major depressive disorders, simple changes to your diet can make a world of difference.

Before we get carried away with the 30 per cent figure, though, let's take a moment to examine the fine print. Participants in this study were supported by seven 60-minute sessions with a dietitian, gifted free food hampers *and* inspired with recipe ideas and motivational interviewing. So, we need to acknowledge that while the dietary change was crucial, the structured support, gifts and professional help were also likely significant contributors to their improvement. Nonetheless, the study is a great example of how comprehensive lifestyle changes – including diet, exercise and mental wellness activities – can all work together to combat depression.

If you were to try the ModiMedDiet, here's a suggestion of what you might eat in a day:

BREAKFAST

A bowl of Greek yoghurt topped with mixed berries and a handful of chopped almonds. You could add a drizzle of honey for some natural sweetness and a sprinkle of chia seeds for extra fibre.

LUNCH

A mixed green salad with grilled chicken, cherry tomatoes, cucumber, red onion, kalamata olives, feta cheese and a simple dressing of olive oil, lemon juice, garlic and oregano.

DINNER

Oven-baked salmon fillet seasoned with lemon, garlic and dill. Serve with cooked quinoa and a side of roasted vegetables, like peppers, courgettes and aubergines, tossed in olive oil and herbs.

SNACKS

Homemade or store-bought hummus served with raw vegetable sticks like carrots, bell peppers or cucumber. You could add a whole-grain pita bread for dipping. Alternatively, you could try some beef jerky for an easy, on-the-go snack that packs high protein, zinc and iron concentrations.

DESSERT

A couple of squares of dark chocolate packed with flavonoids (aim for 70 per cent cocoa or more) served with a selection of your favourite fresh fruits. Ideal fruit choices include berries and citrus fruits.

Tryptophan, B vitamins and folate

Moving on, let's look at another intriguing study that examined the impact of following either a high- or low-tryptophan diet.[19] You might be wondering . . . what's tryptophan? Well, it's an essential amino acid that acts as the building block for serotonin, a neurotransmitter that plays a key role in mood regulation.

In this study, participants experienced fewer depressive symptoms and decreased anxiety while on the tryptophan-rich diet compared to the low-tryptophan diet. Tryptophan cannot be synthesized by the body, so must be obtained through diet. It is especially prevalent in foods like milk, turkey, chicken and canned tuna. In addition to tryptophan, these foods are also rich in B vitamins, which play a similarly key role in preventing and managing depression. Vitamins B1 (thiamine) and B6 (pyridoxine) are important as they help the production of neurotransmitters involved in the regulation of mood. Moreover, a deficiency in vitamin B12 can result in a folate deficiency (vitamin B9) – which can in turn hinder serotonin synthesis and lead to brain-cell death. Depression is the most common symptom of patients with a folate deficiency,[20] and studies show that the higher someone's blood folate level, the lower the severity of their depression.[21]

In summary, tryptophan, B vitamins and folate intakes should be optimized to help prevent and manage depression. Foods that will provide sufficient amounts of all three include lean meats, seafood, chicken, eggs, dairy, legumes, leafy greens, nuts and seeds, as well as fortified foods such as cereals, spreads and nutritional yeast.

Other foods and compounds of interest

FLAVONOIDS

According to new research, flavonoids have potential mood-boosting qualities. These are compounds found in foods like berries, citrus fruits, onions, soybeans, tea, dark chocolate and leafy vegetables. Participants who consumed either flavonoid-rich or low-flavonoid orange juice for eight weeks reported a decrease in depression, hinting at a possible dose-response relationship with flavonoids.[22] Neuroinflammation is one of the main mechanisms involved in the onset of depression, and as we know from the chapter on inflammation, flavonoids are strongly anti-inflammatory in nature.

VITAMIN D OR VITAMIN D3

The active component in blood, vitamin D is an essential component for several physiological functions including muscle performance, bone metabolism, calcium, phosphate homeostasis and our immune system.[23] Vitamin D may be produced via sun exposure or obtained from food, then through two hydroxylation processes in the liver and kidney is converted to vitamin D3.[24] Common food sources include many Mediterranean foods such as salmon, sardines, egg yolk, fortified milk, cereals and yoghurts. Vitamin D has also been shown to be associated with and beneficial for mental health and cognitive function.[25] This is because vitamin D receptors are present in various parts of the brain, including the amygdala, which is responsible for the regulation and balancing of emotions and behaviour. As a result, several studies have found that patients with low vitamin D levels are more likely to suffer from mood disorders.*[26]

MAGNESIUM

Magnesium is crucial for optimal brain functioning as it helps to relay signals between the brain and body, acting as the gatekeeper for the N-methyl-D-aspartate receptors found on nerve cells. These receptors aid brain development and memory.[27] Magnesium-rich foods include nuts, seeds, dry beans, whole grains and green vegetables. Despite being the fourth most abundant mineral in the body, up to 70 per cent of US adults don't meet the recommended daily intake.[28]

The first trial of magnesium treatment for depression was published back in 1921, when it showed a success rate in a massive 220 out of 250 cases! Various case studies exist where patients with major depression were given 125–300mg of magnesium glycinate at each meal and before bed. A rapid improvement in symptoms was noted, often in less than a week.[29] Fast-forward to today, though, and the data is complicated. One meta-analysis of fifty-eight trials covered multiple outcomes, which provided little evidence for the involvement of magnesium in mood disorders like depression.[30]

---

* In a study of 7,970 young adults from the US, they found an 85 per cent increased risk of having depressive episodes if your Vitamin D level was <50nmol/L compared to >75nmol/L. Plenty of controlled trials that have robust methodological design (assessed baseline vitamin D status and given an appropriate dose in the study) have found vitamin D supplementation to be as effective as medication, with the minimum effective dose appearing to be 600–00 IU (international units).

To summarize, the association between magnesium and depression seems plausible, although we don't currently have consistent positive results from human studies. Nonetheless, there are few downsides to consuming a diet rich in magnesium (bearing in mind the upper safety limit of <350mg), and it may help to support good mental health.

SELENIUM

This is an essential mineral that can be found in nuts, seafood, lean meats and whole grains. It's only needed in small amounts but plays an important function in metabolism and thyroid functioning, as well as helping to reduce oxidative stress by minimizing free radical numbers in the blood.[31] Not only is selenium intake associated with improved cognitive function in patients with Alzheimer's disease,[32] it's also been connected to depression. One study found that a low intake of selenium was associated with a threefold increased risk for developing major depressive disorder.[33] Furthermore, intervention trials of selenium supplementation have shown a significant improvement in post-partum depression.[34]

CREATINE

You've all heard of it. Creatine is a substance found naturally in muscle cells that helps in energy utilization. It is also the world's most researched fitness supplement, known for its ability to improve exercise performance, muscle hypertrophy and recovery.[35] Our bodies make around 1g of creatine per day, and it's found in meat, fish and poultry. An untold benefit is its ability to enhance the efficacy and speed by which antidepressants improve depression. Studies in which women with major depressive disorder were given 5g of creatine on top of their SSRI saw a significant improvement in mood compared to the drug alone.[36]

Increasing dietary creatine has been associated with a 32 per cent reduced risk of depression compared to people with the lowest creatine intake. One potential mechanism for how creatine aids in mood is due to its pro-energetic effects in the brain. People with severe depression have abnormal brain bio-energetics (energy-processing in the brain), and creatine improves the regeneration rate of intra-cellular phosphate – which can enhance the effect of SSRIs and potentially improve mood.[37]

SAFFRON

A spice that has historically been widely used to relieve stomach aches and kidney stone pain. In Persian traditional medicine, it was used to treat depression.[38] An analysis of twenty-three controlled trials on saffron supplementation found it had a large positive effect (compared to a placebo) for both depression and anxiety.*[39]

Preclinical studies suggest that saffron contains both crocin and safranal, which have a range of relevant mechanisms. These include antioxidant and anti-inflammatory properties, and an ability to modulate BDNF expression and regulate the hypothalamic–pituitary–axis (HPA). The standard dosage of saffron used in trials is 30mg of saffron (or one drop of powder), with up to 1500mg a day being the safe upper limit. Side effects such as headache, nausea and constipation have been reported, but don't occur at rates greater than placebo or medication groups.

OTHER NUTRIENTS AND COMPOUNDS

Some nutrients and compounds that we don't have time to elaborate on, but have also been shown to play a meaningful role in depression symptomology, include:

- **Iron:** Deficiency (or iron-deficiency anaemia) increases your risk of various psychiatric disorders.[40]

* In the context of standard modern treatments, the results from placebo-controlled trials suggest a superior effect compared to drugs like selective serotonin reuptake inhibitors (SSRIs), although the five trials directly comparing saffron with antidepressants found no statistically significant differences.

- **Curcumin:** The strong antioxidant and anti-inflammatory properties make turmeric (which contains curcumin) ideal to include in your cooking – be sure to add black pepper to increase its bioavailability.[41]
- **Coffee:** Due to its high antioxidant content, combined with caffeine's ability to block adenosine receptors in the brain – reducing fatigue and low mood – dozens of studies show that people who consume higher amounts of coffee have a 24 per cent reduced risk of depression, with the peak protective effect being 400ml/day.[42] That being said, caffeine can exacerbate symptoms of anxiety – especially if you suffer with panic attacks – so if this applies to you then it's probably best to limit your intake.[43]
- **Zinc:** This plays an important role in over 300 biological processes, including DNA replication, maintenance of cell membranes and protein synthesis. It also acts on BDNF and a crucial neurotrophic factor called TrkB, which improves the neuronal connections within the hippocampus.[44] A new meta-analysis showed that the highest levels of zinc intake led to a 28 per cent reduced risk of depression, with zinc supplementation lowering depressive symptoms in depressed patients when used independent of other treatments.[45]

Food for thought

Of course there is no single 'cure' for depression, simply because there is no single *cause* of depression. Like very many health conditions, it is multifactorial in nature. Our internal biology, socio-environmental factors like our living situation and relationships, and lifestyle factors like exercise, diet and sleep all play a role in shaping our mental health. While the field of nutritional psychiatry is expanding exponentially, the current evidence shows that incorporating the above dietary changes can substantially aid in the prevention and treatment of depression outcomes, with few to no negative side effects.*[46]

Now that we've summarized the most important nutrients related to depression, it's time to dive into the science of another debilitating brain disorder: dementia.

Diet and dementia

Dementia is a scary and very serious condition that affects 1 in 14 people over the age of sixty-five in the UK, increasing to 1 in 6 above the age of eighty. It is actually defined as a group of conditions associated with an ongoing decline of brain function, the most prevalent being Alzheimer's disease, which makes up around 70 per cent of dementia cases. Other forms include vascular, frontotemporal and Lewy body dementia.

The more common forms of dementia are characterized by memory loss, reduced thinking speed and difficulty performing daily tasks, as well as a progressive decline in understanding, judgement and movement. Before we jump into the nutrition research, it's important to note that the pathophysiology of dementia is extremely complicated, and there are many factors that play a role in its development and progression. Established risk factors include a family history of the condition, having a lower level of education, high cholesterol or blood pressure,

Fortunately, a lot of the beneficial nutrients we've discussed have been summarized by a massive umbrella review of twenty-eight meta-analyses on the role of dietary factors in the prevention and treatment of depression. The authors analysed studies looking at multiple foods and nutrients. They found that fish consumption and omega-3, zinc, probiotics and coffee lowered your risk of depression. Whereas a pro-inflammatory diet (high DII score), alcohol, low intakes of fruits and veg and the consumption of sugary drinks was associated with a greater risk of depression.

chronic inflammation, insulin resistance, and the usual culprits of smoking and excessive consumption of alcohol, as well as other mental health disorders like depression.

At a cellular level there are two main mechanisms at play in the brain: amyloid plaques, and neurofibrillary tangles that are composed of twisted tau proteins. That probably sounded like a foreign language, but the important thing to understand is that these plaques and proteins can cause a 'neurotoxic cascade' involving neuroinflammation, synaptic dysfunction (in places where neurons connect and interact with each other) and ultimately neuron death. Put simply, more neuron death equals more decline in memory and function. Making effective treatments to halt or prevent these processes has so far been largely unsuccessful.

The roll-out of medication to prevent, delay the onset, slow the progression or improve the symptoms of Alzheimer's disease has proven extremely difficult. In fact, dementia is arguably the most difficult area to treat in all of medicine. The majority of the 244 compounds being tested throughout the 2000s failed to pass the various clinical stages of drug development, with a 99.6 per cent failure rate.[47] As a result of ineffective pharmaceutical interventions, modifiable lifestyle factors – such as nutrition – have taken the research spotlight in the last couple of decades, as we seek to learn more about the prevention and treatment of dementia. So, which foods and compounds have been shown to have an effect on dementia?

Typical Western diets greatly increase dementia risk

While the study of specific nutrients for improving brain health is important in understanding their respective roles in disease states, we don't consume individual nutrients, we consume food. This is why I always say that nutrients do not exist within a vacuum – food is the fundamental unit in nutrition, and research on total dietary patterns provides a basis for whole-diet recommendations. When assessing the diet as a whole, we unfortunately see more and more evidence for the neuron-destructive nature of the Western diet.

The Western-style diet largely comprises pre-packaged ultra-processed foods (UPFs) and meats (think salami and microwave meals), refined grains, red meat, high-sugar drinks, candy, high-fat dairy and fried foods. Worryingly, ultra-processed foods make up 28 per cent of the UK daily diet and form up to 70 per cent of the US food supply! A study of more than 72,000 participants from the UK Biobank cohort followed subjects for an average of ten years.[48] Researchers found that for every 10 per cent increase in daily intake of UPFs, the risk of developing dementia was increased by 25 per cent. Whereas substituting 10 per cent of UPFs with minimally processed foods decreased that risk by 19 per cent. This is likely because UPFs are often high in added sugars, salt and fat, and low in protein and fibre. Additionally, the high level of nitrosamines in processed meats may cause neurodegeneration by impairing the metabolism and signalling mechanisms crucial to brain functionality.[49]

It's also worth thinking about the high glycaemic index (GI) of the Western diet. The brain has a high metabolic rate, and its metabolism is almost entirely dependent on the utilization of glucose. This means that the blood vessels that supply the brain must provide a steady and adequate stream of glucose for optimal functioning. Mounting evidence shows that although an acute rise in blood glucose levels provides some short-term benefits for cognitive performance, a more stable blood-glucose profile, which avoids greater peaks and troughs, is associated with better cognitive function and a lower lifetime risk of cognitive decline.[50] This is why it'd be wise to ensure that most of your meals are sufficiently balanced with unsaturated fats, fibre and protein – all of which slow down digestion and help to maintain a more steady blood-sugar response.

Foods that spike blood sugar rapidly are also associated with greater levels of amyloid burden, which relates to deleterious effects on cognition.[51] This is partly due to an enzyme called insulin degrading enzyme (IDE). IDE is responsible for breaking down insulin (as the name suggests), but also for breaking down amyloid plaques. So, if IDE is busy breaking down lots of insulin from a high-carb/high-GI diet, it has less time to break down amyloid – thus leading to a slow decline in brain power.[52]

The high-GI Western diet can also affect neurons in the hippocampus and prefrontal cortex.[53] The hippocampus is extremely dynamic in that it's heavily involved in our ability to form relational memories – which include remembering facts and events that take place (i.e. recalling new faces, names or facts about the world). So, when you practise remembering things, the hippocampus actually grows. One fascinating study showed that London taxi drivers have much larger posterior hippocampi than other people, as their work involves memorizing vast numbers of streets, routes and landmarks across the city.[54]

However, diets high in refined sugars (and fats) can damage the hippocampus in several different ways. As we discussed earlier in this chapter, refined sugars have been shown to hamper the expression of BDNF in animal models, and BDNF is vital to the healthy functioning of the hippocampus.[55] Furthermore, the high level of saturated fats in the Western diet interferes with cell-signalling pathways and induces insulin resistance, which has been shown to predict cognitive decline in the Tübinger Evaluation of Risk Factors for Early Detection of Neurodegeneration (TREND) study.[56]

Lastly, the Western diet increases oxidative stress, which damages brain tissue and reduces the efficacy of cell-to-cell communication in the hippocampus.[57] This damage can eventually cause it to shrink, which impedes its capacity for memory. This leads to a cascade of negative effects, as the hippocampus is also responsible for regulating how much and what types of foods we eat.

Depression and Dementia

The cycle of refined sugar and fatty diets, and the resulting impact on appetite regulation and brain health, can be difficult to break. High GI, refined sugar and saturated fats summarize the main components of the Western diet that are damaging to the brain.

Dietary advice for dementia

The reality is that the Western diet can nudge us towards dementia, but let's not just focus on what's in it but what's missing too. Next, we'll spotlight the star nutrients and compounds that shield our brains from dementia and introduce you to the ultimate brain-boosting regimen: the MIND diet.

Flavonoids

Flavonoids play an integral part in suppressing systemic inflammation in the body, and given the crucial role of neuroinflammation in dementia, it's clear to see how these compounds provide benefit.[58] It is a little more complicated than this, however. Specific subclasses of flavonoids (anthocyanins and flavonones) have been shown to promote levels of brain-derived neurotrophic factor (BDNF), which as we've just highlighted is crucial for the growth and maturation of neurons.[59] Further to this, flavonoids have been shown to activate an enzyme called endothelial nitric oxide synthase (eNOS), which is responsible for the formation of new blood vessels (angiogenesis) and vasodilation – in turn increasing the amount of blood flow to the brain.[60] This increased blood flow is partly due to BDNF levels being enhanced. Maintaining adequate levels of blood in the brain is crucial, to allow nutrients to reach brain cells and gas exchange to occur.

Eating flavonoid-rich foods has been linked to better cognitive health in multiple observational studies, such as the PAQUID[61] and Nurses' Health studies.[62] In the Nurses' Health study, they found that the consumption of blueberries (>once a week) and strawberries (>twice a week) was associated with a 2.5-year delay in cognitive ageing – meaning that if you were 80 years old, your cognitive ability might be that of a 77-year-old. Generally speaking, higher flavonoid intake is associated with better preservation of cognitive ability and delayed cognitive ageing.

Interventional trials also showed improvements in cognitive function with the consumption of fresh blueberry juice, grape juice and soy products containing isoflavones.[63] One study tested the effects of fresh blueberry juice in healthy adults, and found that word recall and learning were significantly improved after just twelve weeks.[64] Middle-aged working mothers[65] and young children[66] can also benefit from flavonoid-rich diets, as they have been shown to improve performance of everyday tasks and memory.

In summary, incorporating foods high in flavonoids at all stages of life can have significant and long-lasting improvements in terms of cognitive ability.

Fatty fish and omega-3

Omega-3 or fish oil supplements have received some negative press in recent years, due to the latest large-scale review shedding light on their unremarkable effects on cardiovascular health.[67] It turns out that they may not decrease your risk of heart disease to any meaningful degree after all. Separate to that dialogue, there is substantial controversy on whether fish oil benefits brain health – in particular when it comes to memory loss or depression.

There are two parts to this discussion: consuming fatty fish as an actual food, and supplementing with omega-3 or fish oil supplements. In general, the answer is that they can both be beneficial, but let's break down the science to explain why simply reading a research paper won't tell you the whole story.

Fish oil primarily contains two types of omega-3 fatty acids – eicosapentaenoic acid (EPA) and docosahexaenoic acid (DHA). These two fatty acids are important components of cell membranes, and have been implicated in reducing inflammation and aiding the development of a healthy brain and heart. About half of the brain's dry weight is lipid (fat), and around 30 per cent of that is polyunsaturated fatty acids (PUFAs). DHA makes up more than 90 per cent of the omega-3 fats in the brain! This is important because providing the brain with DHA can help divert amyloid proteins away from making amyloid plaques, which cause dementia.[68] Increasing DHA concentrations can also protect the brain from cholesterol-induced amyloid beta production.[69] Finally, both EPA and DHA act as precursors to certain anti-inflammatory compounds known as resolvins (which we touched on in the inflammation chapter), in turn reducing neuro-inflammation crucial for preserving brain function.[70]

In the human diet, EPA and DHA are almost exclusively found in fatty fish and fish oil. Many people fall short of these nutrients as they don't consume two servings of fatty fish per week.[71] The body can make these fatty acids from alpha-linolenic acid, which comes from flaxseed, chia seeds, walnuts and various vegetable oils, however the conversion process from alpha-linolenic acid to EPA/DHA is pretty inefficient, with only 10 per cent of consumed alpha-linolenic acid being converted.[72] Several studies highlight the effectiveness of fatty-fish consumption in protecting against Alzheimer's disease (AD). A meta-analysis of twenty-one studies, including over 181,000 people, looked at their eating habits and followed them for a period of up to twenty-one years.[73] They found that for every one serving of fish consumed per week, the risk of dementia and AD reduced by 5 per cent and 7 per cent respectively.

Some people may try to counter these findings by saying, 'But what about the mercury? It's toxic to the brain.' Let me ease your worries, because the protective effects of fish consumption hold true even when mercury levels are higher in the brain. This is evident from a cross-sectional analysis of the Chicago Memory and Aging Project Study, where people who consumed more fish had higher brain levels of mercury, but still had a massively reduced risk of Alzheimer's disease.[74] Essentially, the benefits of fish consumption far outweigh any possible negatives from mercury contamination.

This is great news! You might then say: 'I'm not really a fan of fish, so I should just pop a couple of omega-3 pills and my brain is good to go, right?' Not so fast . . . The evidence for omega-3 supplementation and AD is entirely inconsistent. Several meta-analyses of controlled interventions show that omega-3 supplements only improve certain aspects of cognitive function in patients with cognitive impairment not associated with dementia.[75] Unremarkable findings were also found in this recent analysis of five controlled trials.[76] There are several reasons why these controlled trials might be so inconsistent. Firstly, the large variability between the dose given to subjects is a problem (it ranged from 240mg to 2.3g per day in one analysis). Furthermore, the duration of each trial was sometimes as little as ninety days, with some being several years. In the context of dementia, those time frames are extremely small. The ratio of DHA to EPA in the supplements was also different. These factors, along with many others, constitute a very significant obstacle when trying to apply results or provide recommendations to people.

So, should we take omega-3 supplements to protect our brain? Despite the lack of consistent intervention trial results due to inconsistencies in study design, the mechanisms and observations across populations are entirely valid. Therefore, people who don't regularly consume fish would likely benefit from regular omega-3 supplementation before a decline in cognition begins.

Rosemary

'There's rosemary, that's for remembrance.' Ophelia, from Shakespeare's *Hamlet*, was on to something. An interesting study in 2012 asked twenty people to sit in cubicles that were infused with the scent of rosemary essential oil, and gave them a variety of cognitive tests in arithmetic, pattern recognition, thinking ability and more.[77] They found that a higher concentration of rosemary was associated with better attention and executive function.

Rosemary has a potent anti-inflammatory capability, through natural oils called diterpenes which protect cells from oxidative stress.[78] Try adding rosemary to roast vegetables, baked potatoes or even on a roasted chicken (a glaze of olive oil will help it to stick). Evidence also shows that the aroma of rosemary can alter brain waves to induce calm, alleviate anxiety and boost alertness.[79]

Coffee

Like rosemary, coffee contains anti-inflammatory diterpenes. Coffee beans also contain many compounds that can be beneficial for brain health. Trigonelline and other polyphenols found in high concentrations within coffee beans can activate antioxidants and protect blood vessels in the brain. On top of its protective effects in terms of depression, coffee is associated with a slower cognitive decline by slowing down amyloid beta accumulation.[80] The caffeine content increases serotonin and acetylcholine, which keeps the brain stimulated and stabilizes the blood brain barrier.

Dozens of trials have demonstrated that caffeine improves energy, mood, attention, reaction time, memory and fatigue in the short term;[81] just remember to keep total caffeine intake below the 400mg/day upper safety limit and avoid it past 3 p.m. to allow optimal sleep.[82]

Irrespective of the effect that coffee has on the brain, its impressive health benefits cannot be ignored. In a very large umbrella review of 201 meta-analyses on coffee and health, with each analysis assessing lots of individual studies, it was found that 3–4 cups of coffee per day saw the greatest reductions in cardiovascular disease, cancer, liver, metabolic disorders and all-cause mortality.[83] Downsides were only seen in pregnancy and the risk of bone fractures for women.

Ginger

Ginger is a powerhouse of a food. It helps to prevent the formation of amyloid plaques and inhibits cholinesterase synthesis – the two main causes for the development of dementia. Due to the beneficial properties observed so far, ginger has actually influenced several studies for the development of new AD drugs.[84] One study found that 400–800mg of ginger extract daily for two months improved working memory significantly in middle-aged women.[85]

The beautiful thing about this magical food is that you can quite literally add ginger to any meal. Muffins with fresh ginger grated on top, curries, marinated meats, cakes, stir-fries . . . you name it, you can add ginger to it.

Vitamin E

Found in nuts, plant-based oils, avocados, seeds and some other fruit and veg, vitamin E is a group of eight fat-soluble compounds. Each sub-form has differing antioxidant activity and acts as a free-radical clean-up crew. Free radicals are unstable and highly reactive molecules produced from normal metabolic processes. In high numbers, they cause damage to organs, cells, proteins and DNA, so it's clear why intaking potent antioxidants like vitamin E can help to protect your brain.

A recent narrative review discussed eleven studies showing some level of neuroprotection from vitamin E in the progression of mild cognitive impairment.[86] However, similar to omega-3 pills, while observations within food have shown great benefit, supplemental vitamin E studies have proven unsuccessful due to supplements using different compositions of tocopherols, which may be ineffective.[87]

Calorie restriction

It's worth mentioning calorie restriction briefly. With the modern food environment we live in today, generally people are over-consuming rather than under-consuming food, and because of the negative implications of overeating on inflammation it's not surprising to see strong evidence for the benefits of calorie restriction on cognitive and brain health. In 2019, researchers conducted a clinical trial as part of the larger CALERIE study, comparing working memory in healthy middle-aged adults who restricted their calories by 25 per cent over two years with a control group who consumed as much as they wanted.[88] They found a significant improvement in working memory in those who calorie-restricted, which held true after accounting for sleep quality and exercise.

These findings are solidified by a brand-new meta-analysis of eleven controlled trials which showed that calorie restriction through normal methods or intermittent fasting resulted in varying degrees of positive effect on cognitive function in overweight and normal-weighted individuals.[89] However it's important to note that this doesn't necessarily apply to all populations. If you're someone who doesn't eat much to begin with or lacks adequate intake of nutrient-rich foods, then you may not be benefitting your brain by further restricting calorie intake. With decisions like this, it's important to consult your doctor to find a suitable plan for you.

The MIND diet

As the name suggests, the MIND (or Mediterranean-DASH Intervention for Neurodegenerative Delay) diet was designed by nutritional epidemiologist Martha Clare Morris specifically to prevent dementia and the loss of brain function as a result of ageing. It comprises a dietary concoction of foods and nutrients specifically tailored to support brain health. In 2015, Dr Morris compiled a list of dietary components that were either positive or negative for cognition. She highlighted ten brain-healthful food groups for the MIND diet, as follows:

- Green, leafy vegetables (such as kale, spinach or cooked greens)
- Other vegetables (broccoli, carrots, peppers, non-starchy vegetables)
- Berries (blueberries, strawberries, raspberries, blackberries)
- Nuts
- Beans
- Olive oil
- Whole grains
- Fish
- Poultry
- 1 glass wine*[90]

---

* However, it's becoming clearer as the years go by that there really is no 'safe' limit of alcohol consumption even for the brain, which is contradictory to the recommendations of the MIND diet. Heavy alcohol consumption has been linked to brain atrophy, neuronal loss and poorer white matter fibres, which are the nerve extensions crucial in transmitting brain impulses. Research from the UK Biobank cohort where they medically imaged 36,678 brains demonstrates that even people who consume 1–2 units of alcohol a day (a single drink) have reduced brain volumes and poorer white-matter microstructure. Therefore, despite what some people may tell you about compounds in wine

This was accompanied by five brain-damaging food groups:

- Red meat
- Margarine and butter
- Cheese
- Pastries
- Sweets and fried/ultra-processed fast foods

The Memory and Aging Project study, which assessed residents from more than forty retirement communities in Chicago, nicely demonstrates the benefits of the MIND diet. Dr Morris and her colleagues assigned a diet score to each of the food types, so they could assess how well subjects were sticking to the diet. Take the leafy green vegetable category, for example. The optimal MIND score for that category of food is six or more servings per week. If a participant consumed fewer than two servings per week that would score 0; between two and six servings per week would score 0.5; and 1 point could be earned for eating more than six servings per week. For the harmful food groups, the scoring system is simply reversed – so consuming more than seven or more servings of red meat per week would score 0 points, between four and six servings would score 0.5, and less than four servings per week would score 1 point.

The participants' dietary habits were analysed and MIND diet scores that reflected their level of adherence were allocated. The fascinating finding was that those with the highest MIND scores were 7.5 years younger in cognitive age than those with the lowest scores.[91] These associations stood strong for total cognitive score, but also for each of the five domains of cognitive health: semantic memory (memory of facts and general world knowledge), working memory (short-term recall of information that is being acted upon), perceptual speed (how fast things are seen), visuospatial

_____

uch as resveratrol being brain-boosting, you're simply better off just not consuming alcohol, for a whole host of reasons.

ability (the ability to see and comprehend the size and space of the environment) and episodic memory (long-term recall of information that is still being acted upon). Interestingly, the greatest benefits were seen in episodic memory, semantic memory and perceptual speed. The MIND diet was also associated with a reduced risk of Alzheimer's disease.

Since Martha's initial study, there have been a plethora of trials which support her findings. In 2019, a study in Australia also found that the MIND diet was linked to a reduced risk of Alzheimer's disease over a twelve-year follow-up period.[92] And a recent systematic review of thirteen studies indicates that adherence to the MIND diet is positively associated with specific domains of cognitive performance in older adults. Perhaps most importantly, though, the MIND diet has been shown to be superior to other plant-rich diets including the MD, DASH and Pro-Vegetarian diets for improving cognition.[93]

In summary, the MIND diet seems to provide the best foundation for the protection of memory and cognitive decline. It's probably wise to integrate as many of these dietary components as you can into your daily routine. Below is a summary of the main principles:

The 10 brain-healthful food groups based on the MIND diet (each scores 1 point)	
Green leafy vegetables (kale, chard, spinach, cooked greens and green salad)	6 or more servings per week
Other vegetables (peppers, carrots, broccoli, potatoes, peas, celery, tomatoes, string beans, beetroot, corn, aubergine, etc.)	1 or more servings per day

Berries (blueberries, raspberries, blackberries, strawberries)	2 or more servings per week
Olive oil	Primary oil source
Nuts	5 or more servings per week
Whole grains	3 or more servings per week
Fish (fatty fish high in omega-3, e.g. salmon)	1 or more servings per week
Beans (lentils, soybeans, generic beans)	More than 3 servings per week
Poultry (chicken or turkey)	2 or more servings per week
Wine	1 glass per day

Remember that these are the optimal dietary principles of the MIND diet. It doesn't really matter if you can't follow all of them; research still shows that following the MIND diet even slightly is associated with a reduced risk of Alzheimer's disease.

Key takeaways

1. **Lower your glycaemic load.** Constant peaks and troughs in blood sugar levels through excessive refined-sugar intake can affect your mood, increase your risk of depression and affect your short -and long-term cognitive health. The brain functions optimally with a steady stream of glucose and nutrients; therefore, focusing on complex carbohydrates like whole grains, as well as unsaturated fats, fibre and protein with most meals, will lower the GI tremendously. Not to mention

that this principle for a main meal will aid in appetite, calorie intake and cravings throughout the day.

2. **Calorie restriction.** If you're overweight (which means you have been overconsuming food for a prolonged period of time), one of the best things you can do to protect your brain is to reduce the number of calories you're consuming. This can often be achieved indirectly by focusing on the MIND and ModiMedDiet recommendations. Taking on board the detailed strategies and solutions to sustainably reduce calories from the weight-loss chapter will also serve you well.

3. **Season your food!** Saffron, turmeric, ginger, rosemary and various chillies with anti-inflammatory properties are easy and tasty non-caloric additions to your everyday diet which can make a huge difference to your brain and mental health. Some of these ingredients (in appropriate dosages) are as effective as some antidepressant medications.

4. **Engage with the values of the MIND and ModiMedDiet** (with the exception of wine intake). These are based on specified dietary principles specifically developed to improve your mood and protect your brain.

5. **Don't inflame your brain!** Neuroinflammation is one of the main players in cognitive and mental decline, so following the principles of the inflammation chapter (i.e. an 'anti-inflammatory' dietary pattern) is crucial for long-term brain health.

Concluding Thoughts

As we bring our journey of myth-busting and truth-seeking to close, it is my sincerest hope that you, the reader, feel not just informed but also empowered. The world of nutrition is an ever-evolving landscape – a complex mosaic of theories, studies and recommendations, each one clamouring for our attention and belief. Yet, amid this cacophony of information, you now wield the tools to sift fact from fiction and evidence from exaggeration.

In debunking the myths that have so long clouded our understanding of nutrition, we have laid bare the simple, universal truth: there are no magic bullets, no one-size-fits-all diets, no secrets to instantaneous health and wellness. A journey towards healthier living is typically a series of small, manageable and sustainable lifestyle choices, guided by reliable information and personal introspection.

As you move forward, remember that the path to wellness is not a sprint, but a marathon. Nutrition and health are not about strict restrictions, crash diets or quick fixes. They're about balance, variety and moderation. Eating a rainbow of fruits and vegetables, getting enough protein and hydrating adequately are all more effective and scientifically supported than any fad diet or so-called superfood.

In this book, we have dismantled many nutrition myths, from the foolishness of miracle weight-loss remedies to the demonization of carbohydrates and the glorification of certain foods as miracle cures. Yet it is inevitable that new myths will continue to emerge, armed with compelling narratives and alluring promises. Our most potent defence remains your ability to think critically.

Always remember to question the source of information, scrutinize the evidence, and seek out expert opinions when in doubt. In an age when misinformation can spread like wildfire, this mindset is your extinguisher.

We can take solace in the increasing number of doctors, dietitians and health professionals dedicated to combating misinformation and promoting fact-based nutritional and health advice. Moreover, governments, non-profit organizations and even some media outlets are implementing stricter regulations and fact-checking mechanisms to stem the tide of health misinformation. Keep in mind that it is okay to make mistakes and learn as you go. Each debunked myth, each corrected misconception, brings you one step closer to understanding the intricate puzzle that is human nutrition. So, embrace the journey with curiosity and an open mind.

The world of nutrition may seem like a labyrinth of conflicting information, but you are no hapless wanderer. You are an informed navigator, armed with a compass of scientific literacy. As you chart your course towards better health, remember to be patient with yourself, stay curious and always maintain a healthy dose of scepticism. You now have the power to explore the frontiers of your health, to make informed decisions and, most importantly, to champion your well-being. In that spirit, let's step forward – not with trepidation, but with optimism – towards a healthier, brighter future.

After all, you are the author of your own health story. Make it a tale worth telling.

Appendix
Hierarchy of Evidence

One can find a research paper to support any view. I've had count-less interactions with influencers saying that they've done their 'research'. But let me ask you, what does 'doing your research' actually mean? For a lot of people it means asking Google and finding the first tabloid article on the topic. For others it means typing 'carbs cause weight gain' into a research database and seeing what pops up. Neither of these methods is classified as 'doing research'. The distinguishing factor here is that I use my expertise in critical appraisal to condense and summarize compli-cated and nuanced scientific topics.

With this in mind, it's a good idea to mention that not all stud-ies are equal, so let's briefly run through the different types of research studies, exploring their strengths and limitations.

Hierarchy of evidence	Description	Strengths	Limitations
Meta-analysis / systematic review	A robust analysis of multiple studies on the same topic – to give you an unbiased overview of the best available evidence (a study on studies).	The strongest type of scientific evidence.	Its strength depends on the quality of the available evidence (i.e. an analysis of poorly designed studies won't yield strong conclusions).
Literature review	Researchers provide an overview of the available evidence on any given topic – without any formal method of reviewing. (E.g. Does dairy consumption affect cardiovascular disease risk?)	Gives you a good foundational understanding for any given topic which utilizes the available evidence of that time. (A 2017 literature review will only provide insight into the evidence before 2017.)	As it doesn't follow rigorous or transparent methods for the review process, we cannot call it a systematic review and therefore it doesn't hold the same weight. Subject to author bias (the author decides which studies they discuss).

Randomized controlled trial (RCT)	Researchers recruit a group of people and directly test the effect of an intervention on an aspect of health (e.g. testing the effect of consuming high-fructose corn syrup on inflammatory blood markers).	Directly tests the effects of an intervention by comparing it to a placebo or 'control' group. Controls for more variables compared to observational research. Provides evidence for 'cause and effect'.	Findings can only be applied to the demographic that was tested (e.g. a study on 40- to 50-year-old women can't be applied to young men). Often short-term and expensive. Not able to test many hypotheses due to ethical reasons.

Appendix

Observational studies	Researchers monitor and observe large groups of people and analyse associations between certain lifestyle choices. (E.g. Do those who eat more red meat get more colorectal cancer?)	Allows us to predict the risk of disease from a lifestyle habit over many years. Often looks at entire populations which can be sub-grouped to see the impact on different demographics such as ages/genders/health status, etc. Provides the grounds to conduct RCTs.	Unable to control confounding variables as strongly as an RCT. Provides us with associations and not causations. (NOT always the case! See page 191.)
Animal studies	Testing the effect of a food or nutrient on a group of animals (usually rats).	Findings allow us to better understand the potential impact of an intervention on humans.	Findings cannot be applied to humans until strong human evidence confirms it.

		Findings allow us to better understand the potential impact of an intervention on humans.	Findings cannot be applied to humans until full-body human evidence confirms it.
In vitro studies	Testing the effect of a food or nutrient on a collection of human cells or tissue.		
Expert opinion	A qualified expert in the field giving their rationale or hypothesis based on their knowledge and experience without citing relevant research. ('I think that high insulin levels may affect weight loss.')	Far more credible than a simple anecdote from a layperson.	Not classified as objective evidence.
Anecdote	Any individual recalling their own experiences. ('The only thing that worked for me was cutting out sugar, therefore you have to cut sugar out to lose weight.')	No strengths.	Not classified as objective evidence.

Appendix

Observational vs controlled research

Nutritional research is largely based on observational data. This is arguably the most valuable part of nutrition research and I'll explain why.

Based on the hierarchy of evidence above, it's clear to see that randomized controlled trials would be more valuable, no? Well, it's not actually that simple. When talking about chronic diseases like cardiovascular disease, type 2 diabetes and fatty liver disease, these things don't just happen in a few weeks. They occur over decades of lifestyle, environmental and genetic influences. Say you wanted to see if refined sugars *cause* diabetes over time. You'd need to design an RCT whereby one group of young adults is given a large amount of refined (or added) sugar every day while another group is not, keeping all their other foods the same. The groups would need to be monitored, have their activity levels controlled, and a record would need to be kept of every single food they'd eaten for at least twenty years. Does this sound ethical to you? Most definitely not. The long-term health implications of excess refined sugar intake are pretty clear in the literature. This dietary habit drastically increases your risk of obesity, cardiovascular disease, diabetes and even some cancers. Therefore, by conducting a study like this, you'd be intentionally causing harm to people. Not only that, but supervising and managing a study of this length – and waiting two decades to have the data for a singular study – would be extremely costly, both financially and in relation to time. This is why, when assessing disease risk from specific nutrients or foods in the diet, it is almost always from observational data where large groups of people have been observed (not forced to act a certain way), and that data is then analysed to find trends between dietary habits and disease prevalence.

Now, that being said, RCTs do still have an important role in nutrition and health. Let's take the refined sugar example once more. We can test for acute changes in things like biochemical and inflammatory blood markers. We could test the effect of refined sugars on our insulin levels, insulin resistance and blood sugar levels. If the level of insulin resistance in our cells went up over four weeks, we could then hypothesize that this would cause type 2 diabetes over time – as we know that insulin resistance is a key driver in the aetiology (cause) of diabetes. But this is only scientifically appropriate if it's supported by large-scale observational data over many years, showing that diets high in refined sugar are more likely to lead to diabetes in the future. This is a key component in how to appropriately apply the evidence base of a topic.

Just to make it clear, I'm not saying that sugar is inherently harmful in any amount. It's far more nuanced than that. I'm simply walking you through an example and how to draw appropriate conclusions.

Another aspect of observational data that most people don't quite understand is that correlation *can* actually mean causation. Perhaps you are thinking that doesn't sound right. Well, let's talk through the example of smoking and lung cancer. It's common knowledge that smoking is a direct cause of cancer but there is not a single RCT showing that smoking causes cancer, so how can that be right? Of course there isn't, because once again how on earth can you force a group of people to smoke for twenty years until some of them get cancer? We aren't lab rats, and nor would we even be able to treat people like lab rats. Life is *not* controlled, and we all make our own decisions.

The reason we are able to classify smoking as a 'cause' of cancer is because the level of observational evidence we have is extremely robust. These findings have been replicated across many different populations, have been repeated with little evidence showing the opposite, have plausible biological mechanisms that are well established, and the effect sizes are clinically relevant (meaning the increase in disease risk is meaningful). These are some of the criteria for upgrading an association from correlation to causation.

This is why assessing both the observational and interventional data is particularly profound. Too many people who may not understand research in depth are sceptical of results if they don't originate from an RCT. 'Correlation is not causation' is a typical comment I find in my videos. However, because of the factors explained above, I'd argue that nutrition is one of the few scientific fields whereby observational data actually provides more value than RCTs.

Industry-funded research

I have received thousands of comments and had countless interactions with people simply dismissing scientific evidence because some of the studies are 'funded by industry'. This is a classic rebuttal when the evidence undermines one's own hypothesis or held biases, and is most often seen when discussing the health effects of pharmaceuticals, meat or dairy. Now, while it's true that financial conflicts of interest can influence research, it is entirely inappropriate to dismiss evidence simply because of this reason.

There are several complex reasons why research funding doesn't tell us the whole story, but possibly the simplest to understand is that publishing health research in journals has many procedures in place that minimize the influence of industry. This is particularly true for most biomedical research journals, which now require prior registration of clinical trials in a public database as a condition of publication. This means the researchers must provide the aims, objectives, analysis, methods, research sites and investigators all before their findings are published. On top of this, plenty of journals like the *Journal of the American*

Medical Association (JAMA) require the data analysis for industry-funded studies to be conducted by an independent statistician at an academic institution rather than an employee of the company.[1] They also require one author who is independent of the sponsor to have full access to all of the data, and they then take responsibility for data analysis and accuracy.

Furthermore, researchers who have received funding from industry can sign agreements that, regardless of what the results show, they will publish it. Procedures like this apply to many prestigious research journals, which makes it difficult to manipulate data. People who don't trust industry-funded research are forgetting that government-funded studies can also have agendas, such as a political motivation to conduct a study. Therefore, it's extremely naive to dismiss other forms of bias when we have plenty of scientific reviews discussing the impacts of 'non-financial conflicts of interest'. This is why 'who funded it' is not a reliable indicator of validity.

Journals tend to be more interested in research data with lower p values ($p < 0.05$), meaning that we're more than 95 per cent certain the results are not due to chance, because it shows a stronger effect or association. Private organizations have the capacity to invest and conduct clinical trials of a larger scale and sample size. This means that the statistical power of a study is increased and therefore is more likely to detect a difference between treatments (i.e. positive results). Thus, the amount of funding available for research may skew the publication record in favour of industry-funded studies without evidence of foul play.

Notably, if private funders have exciting preliminary evidence that a product is shown to be particularly effective, they are far more inclined to fund additional trials for that product. For example, companies could run a pilot study (small-scale) to begin with and, based on those findings, could then choose to conduct a larger identical study if those results are exciting. This also means that a company could decide against funding a study based on the preliminary evidence due to lack of effectiveness. Decisions like these create associations between financial interests and research outcomes that have little to do with dishonesty or malfeasance.

The next crucial point is that government-funded studies do not have millions of pounds to spend on large randomized controlled trials, so the larger, more influential studies will likely have to be funded by private corporations. Therefore, in certain scientific fields there will be a natural skew towards industry-funded research – such as in the pharmaceutical, meat and dairy industries. This has nothing to do with manipulation of data, it's simply a cost issue. And there are other, more complex reasons why you shouldn't simply dismiss industry-funded research, such as the difficulty in manipulating research data, the type of statistical tests you use and the type of study it is. For example, meta-analyses of controlled studies are harder to manipulate than complex longitudinal studies with masses of variable data. This is why remaining objective and not letting the funding source influence your analysis is wise. One study assessing the effect of disclosing authors' conflict-of-interest declarations to peer reviewers at a medical journal is a perfect example of this. They found that regardless of whether the author of a study had a conflict of interest or not, this did not affect the mean quality rating of each study.[2]

The point is: focusing on the fact that a study is industry-funded often results in an unreliable assessment of its validity. You could have a perfectly well-designed meta-analysis of forty-three controlled studies, but just because it's funded by a corporation that has no role in how the study is carried out, you simply dismiss it. What this allows people to do is to completely disregard any evidence that doesn't fit their bias, and to hold beliefs that aren't backed by strong scientific literature. This is confirmation bias. Instead, we should assess the scientific merit of a study, take all the evidence as a whole and not worry too much about how it was funded.

Acknowledgements

Immense gratitude to Ms Laura Roberts (surgeon) for bestowing this book with its title, to Dr Hannah Reilly for helping to organize my thoughts in the early stages of writing and to Drs Alisha Pradhan and Mini Kharel, whose belief in me breathed life into my online platform and, in turn, this very book.

Notes

Introduction

1 Statista Research Department, 'Share of Individuals in the United Kingdom seeking health information online from 2009 to 2020', 8 August 2023, https://www.statista.com/statistics/1236817/united-kingdom-internet-users-seeking-health-information-online/.

2 G. Eysenbach et al., 'Empirical studies assessing the quality of health information for consumers on the World Wide Web: A systematic review', *JAMA*, 287(20), 2002, pp. 2691–700, https://doi.org/10.1001/jama.287.20.2691.

3 K. S. Hall et al., 'Systematic review of the prospective association of daily step counts with risk of mortality, cardiovascular disease, and dysglycemia', *International Journal of Behavioral Nutrition and Physical Act*, 17(1), 2020, article 78, https://doi.org/10.1186/s12966-020-00978-9.

Truth and Lies

1 I. D'Andrea Meira et al., 'Ketogenic diet and epilepsy: What we know so far', *Frontiers in Neuroscience*, 13, 29 January 2019, p. 5, https://doi.org/10.3389/fnins.2019.00005.

2 K. D. Hall et al., 'Calorie for calorie, dietary fat restriction results in more body fat loss than carbohydrate restriction in people with obesity', *Cell Metabolism*, 22(3), September 2015, pp. 427–36, https://doi.org/10.1016/j.cmet.2015.07.021; K. D. Hall et al., 'Energy expenditure and body composition changes after an isocaloric ketogenic diet in

overweight and obese men', *American Journal of Clinical Nutrition*, 104(2), August 2016, pp. 324–33, https://doi.org/10.3945/ajcn.116.133561.

3 D. S. Ludwig and C. B. Ebbeling, 'The carbohydrate-insulin model of obesity: Beyond "calories in, calories out"', *JAMA Internal Medicine*, 178(8), August 2018, pp. 1098–1103, https://doi.org/10.1001/jamainternmed.2018.2933.

4 E. A. Spencer et al., 'Diet and body mass index in 38000 EPIC-Oxford meat-eaters, fish-eaters, vegetarians and vegans', *International Journal of Obesity and Related Metabolic Disorders*, 27(6), June 2003, pp. 728–34, https://doi.org/10.1038/sj.ijo.0802300.

5 J. S. Dybvik et al., 'Vegetarian and vegan diets and the risk of cardiovascular disease, ischemic heart disease and stroke: A systematic review and meta-analysis of prospective cohort studies', *European Journal of Nutrition*, 27 August 2022, pp. 51–69, https://doi.org/10.1007/s00394-022-02942-8.

6 D. Buettner and S. Skemp, 'Blue Zones: Lessons from the world's longest-lived', *American Journal of Lifestyle Medicine*, 10(5), July 2016, pp. 318–21, https://doi.org/10.1177/1559827616637066.

7 O. T. Mytton et al., 'Systematic review and meta-analysis of the effect of increased vegetable and fruit consumption on body weight and energy intake', *BMC Public Health*, 14(1), August 2014, p. 886, https://doi.org/10.1186/1471-2458-14-886; erratum in *BMC Public Health*, 17(1), August 2017, p. 662.

8 K. C. Maki et al., 'The Relationship between whole grain intake and body weight: Results of meta-analyses of observational studies and randomized controlled trials', *Nutrients*, 11(6), May 2019, p. 1245, https://doi.org/10.3390/nu11061245.

9 S. J. Kim et al., 'Effects of dietary pulse consumption on body weight: A systematic review and meta-analysis of randomized controlled trials', *American Journal of Clinical Nutrition*, 103(5), May 2016, pp. 1213–23, https://doi.org/10.3945/ajcn.115.124677.

10 Y. J. Choi et al., 'Impact of a ketogenic diet on metabolic parameters in patients with obesity or overweight and with or without type 2

Notes

diabetes: A meta-analysis of randomized controlled trials', *Nutrients*, 12(7), July 2020, https://doi.org/10.3390/nu12072005.

11 J. T. Batch et al., 'Advantages and disadvantages of the ketogenic diet: A review article', *Cureus*, 12(8), August 2020, e9639, https://doi.org/10.7759/cureus.9639.

12 J. B. Calton, 'Prevalence of micronutrient deficiency in popular diet plans', *Journal of the International Society of Sports Nutrition*, 7(1), June 2010, article 24, https://doi.org/10.1186/1550-2783-7-24.

13 J. Burén et al., 'A ketogenic low-carbohydrate high-fat diet increases LDL cholesterol in healthy, young, normal-weight women: A randomized controlled feeding trial', *Nutrients*, 13(3), March 2021, p. 814, https://doi.org/10.3390/nu13030814.

14 B. A. Ference et al., 'Low-density lipoproteins cause atherosclerotic cardiovascular disease. 1. Evidence from genetic, epidemiologic, and clinical studies. A consensus statement from the European Atherosclerosis Society Consensus Panel', *European Heart Journal*, 38(32), 2017, pp. 2459–72, https://doi.org/10.1093/eurheartj/ehx144.

15 M. Mazidi et al., 'Lower carbohydrate diets and all-cause and cause-specific mortality: A population-based cohort study and pooling of prospective studies', *European Heart Journal*, 40(34), September 2019, pp. 2870–9, https://doi.org/10.1093/eurheartj/ehz174.

16 X. Wei, 'Intermittent Energy Restriction for Weight Loss: A Systematic Review of Cardiometabolic, Inflammatory and Appetite Outcomes', *Biological Research for Nursing*, 24(3), 2022, pp. 410–28, https://doi.org/10.1177/10998004221078079; L. Gu, 'Effects of Intermittent Fasting in Human Compared to a Non-intervention Diet and Caloric Restriction: A Meta-Analysis of Randomized Controlled Trials', *Frontiers in Nutrition*, 9, 2022, 871682, https://doi.org/10.3389/fnut.2022.871682.

17 E. F. Sutton et al., 'Early time-restricted feeding improves insulin sensitivity, blood pressure, and oxidative stress even without weight loss in men with prediabetes', *Cell Metabolism*, 27(6), June 2018, pp. 1212–21.e3, https://doi.org/10.1016/j.cmet.2018.04.010.

18 F. Antunes et al., 'Autophagy and intermittent fasting: the connec tion for cancer therapy?' *Clinics* (Sao Paulo), December 2018, 10;73(1) e814s, https://doi.org/10.6061/clinics/2018/e814s.

19 C. W. Cheng et al., 'Prolonged fasting reduces IGF-1/PKA to pro mote hematopoietic-stem-cell-based regeneration and reverse immunosuppression', *Cell Stem Cell*, 14(6), June 2014, pp. 810–23 https://doi.org/10.1016/j.stem.2014.04.014. Erratum in: *Cell Stem Cell*, 18(2), February 2018, pp. 291–2.

20 L. Fontana et al., 'Long-term effects of calorie or protein restriction on serum IGF-1 and IGFBP-3 concentration in humans', *Aging Cell*, 7(5), October 2008, pp. 681–7, https://doi.org/10.1111/j.1474 9726.2008.00417.x.

21 K. K. Clifton et al., 'Intermittent fasting in the prevention and treat ment of cancer', *CA: A Cancer Journal for Clinicians*, 71(6), Novembe 2021, pp. 527–46, https://doi.org/10.3322/caac.21694.

22 K. Cuccolo et al., 'Intermittent fasting implementation and assoc ation with eating disorder symptomatology', *Eating Disorder* September–October 2022, 30(5), pp. 471–91, https://doi.org/10.1080 10640266.2021.1922145.

23 Precedence Research, 'Vegan Food Market', https://www precedenceresearch.com/vegan-food-market.

24 J. R. Benatar and R. A. H. Stewart, 'Cardiometabolic risk factors i vegans: A meta-analysis of observational studies', *PLoS One*, 13(12 December 2018, e0209086, https://doi.org/10.1371/journal.pone 0209086.

25 J. Quek et al., 'The Association of Plant-Based Diet with Cardio vascular Disease and Mortality: A Meta-Analysis and System atic Review of Prospect Cohort Studies', *Frontiers in Cardiovascula Medicine*, 8, November 2021, https://doi.org/10.3389/fcvm.202 756810.

26 D. Rogerson et al., 'Contrasting Effects of Short-Term Mediterra nean and Vegan Diets on Microvascular Function and Cholester in Younger Adults: A Comparative Pilot Study', *Nutrients*, 10(12 December 2018, p. 1897, https://doi.org/10.3390/nu10121897.

27 F. Sofi et al., 'Low-Calorie Vegetarian Versus Mediterranean Diets for Reducing Body Weight and Improving Cardiovascular Risk Profile: CARDIVEG Study (Cardiovascular Prevention With Vegetarian Diet)', *Circulation*, 137(11), March 2018, pp. 1103–13, https://doi.org/10.1161/CIRCULATIONAHA.117.030088.

28 R. Pawlak et al., 'The prevalence of cobalamin deficiency among vegetarians assessed by serum vitamin B12: a review of literature', *European Journal of Clinical Nutrition*, 68(5), May 2014, pp. 541–8, https://doi.org/10.1038/ejcn.2014.46. Erratum in: *European Journal of Clinical Nutrition*, 70(7), July 2016, p. 866.

29 R. Pawlak et al., 'Iron Status of Vegetarian Adults: A Review of Literature', *American Journal of Lifestyle Medicine*, 12(6), December 2016, pp. 486–98, https://doi.org/10.1177/1559827616682933.

30 D. Skolmowska and D. Głąbska, 'Analysis of Heme and Non-Heme Iron Intake and Iron Dietary Sources in Adolescent Menstruating Females in a National Polish Sample', *Nutrients*, 11(5), May 2019, pp. 1049, https://doi.org/10.3390/nu11051049.

31 T. A. Sanders, 'Growth and development of British vegan children', *American Journal of Clinical Nutrition*, 48(3), September 1988, p. 822–5, https://doi.org/10.1093/ajcn/48.3.822.

32 M. A. O'Connor et al., 'Vegetarianism in anorexia nervosa? A review of 116 consecutive cases', *Medical Journal of Australia*, 147(11–12), December 1987, pp. 540–2, https://doi.org/10.5694/j.1326-5377.1987.tb133677.x.

33 A. M. Bardone-Cone et al., 'The inter-relationships between vegetarianism and eating disorders among females', *Journal of the Academy of Nutrition and Dietetics*, 112(8), August 2012, pp. 1247–52, https://doi.org/10.1016/j.jand.2012.05.007.

34 I. Berrazaga et al., 'The Role of the Anabolic Properties of Plant- versus Animal-Based Protein Sources in Supporting Muscle Mass Maintenance: A Critical Review', *Nutrients*, 11(8), August 2019, p. 1825, https://doi.org/10.3390/nu11081825.

35 P. J. Garlick, 'The role of leucine in the regulation of protein metabolism', *Journal of Nutrition*, 135(6), June 2005, pp. 1553S–6S, https://doi.org/10.1093/jn/135.6.1553S.

36 V. Hevia-Larraín et al., 'High-Protein Plant-Based Diet Versus a Protein-Matched Omnivorous Diet to Support Resistance Training Adaptations: A Comparison Between Habitual Vegans and Omnivores', *Sports Medicine*, 51(6), June 2021, pp. 1317–30, https://doi.org/10.1007/s40279-021-01434-9.

37 L. Herreman et al., 'Comprehensive overview of the quality of plant- and animal-sourced proteins based on the digestible indispensable amino acid score', *Food Science & Nutrition*, 8, 2020, pp. 5379–91, https://doi.org/10.1002/fsn3.1809.

38 J. Poore and T. Nemecek, 'Reducing food's environmental impacts through producers and consumers', *Science*, 360(6392), 1 June 2018, pp. 987–92, https://doi.org/10.1126/science.aaq0216. Erratum in: *Science*, 363(6429), February 2019.

39 A. Shepon et al., 'Energy and protein feed-to-food conversion efficiencies in the US and potential food security gains from dietary changes', *Environmental Research Letters*, 11(10), 2018, 105002, https://doi.org/10.1088/1748-9326/11/10/105002.

40 R. Wang and S. Guo, 'Phytic acid and its interactions: Contributions to protein functionality, food processing, and safety', *Comprehensive Reviews in Food Science and Food Safety*, 20(2), March 2021, pp. 2081–2105, https://doi.org/10.1111/1541-4337.12714.

41 L. Shi et al., 'Changes in levels of phytic acid, lectins and oxalates during soaking and cooking of Canadian pulses', *Food Research International*, 107, May 2018, pp. 660–8, https://doi.org/10.1016/j.foodres.2018.02.056.

42 A. Kumar et al., 'Phytic acid: Blessing in disguise, a prime compound required for both plant and human nutrition', *Food Research International*, 142, April 2021, article 110193, https://doi.org/10.1016/j.foodres.2021.110193.

43 E. B. Nchanji and O. C. Ageyo, 'Do Common Beans (*Phaseolus vulgaris* L.) Promote Good Health in Humans? A Systematic Review and Meta-Analysis of Clinical and Randomized Controlled Trials', *Nutrients*, 13(11), October 2021, p. 3701, https://doi.org/10.3390/nu13113701.

44 Z. Y. Liu et al., 'Trimethylamine N-oxide, a gut microbiota-dependent metabolite of choline, is positively associated with the risk of primary liver cancer: a case-control study', *Nutrition & Metabolism*, 15, November 2018, p. 81, https://doi.org/10.1186/s12986-018-0319-2.

45 V. Fiorito et al., 'The Multifaceted Role of Heme in Cancer', *Frontiers in Oncology*, 9, January 2020, p. 1540, https://doi.org/10.3389/fonc.2019.01540.

46 M. Khazaei, 'Chronic Low-grade Inflammation after Exercise: Controversies', *Iranian Journal of Basic Medical Sciences*, 15(5), September 2012, pp. 1008–9, https://pubmed.ncbi.nlm.nih.gov/23495361.

47 H. Okada et al., 'The "hygiene hypothesis" for autoimmune and allergic diseases: An update', *Clinical & Experimental Immunology*, 160(1), April 2010, pp. 1–9, https://doi.org/10.1111/j.1365-2249.2010.04139.x.

48 T. C. Wallace et al., 'Fruits, vegetables, and health: A comprehensive narrative, umbrella review of the science and recommendations for enhanced public policy to improve intake', *Critical Reviews in Food Science and Nutrition*, 60(13), 2020, pp. 2174–2211, https://doi.org/10.1080/10408398.2019.1632258.

49 N. F. Aykan, 'Red Meat and Colorectal Cancer', *Oncology Reviews*, 9(1), December 2015, p. 288, https://doi.org/10.4081/oncol.2015.288.

50 L. Hooper et al., 'Reduction in saturated fat intake for cardiovascular disease', *Cochrane Database of Systematic Reviews*, 5(5), May 2020, CD011737, https://doi.org/10.1002/14651858.CD011737.pub2.

51 N. Becerra-Tomás et al., 'Mediterranean diet, cardiovascular disease and mortality in diabetes: A systematic review and meta-analysis of prospective cohort studies and randomized clinical trials', *Critical Reviews in Food Science and Nutrition*, 60(7), 2020, pp. 1207–27, https://doi.org/10.1080/10408398.2019.1565281.

52 K. Esposito et al., 'Mediterranean diet and weight loss: meta-analysis of randomized controlled trials', *Metabolic Syndrome and Related Disorders*, 9(1), February 2011, pp. 1–12, https://doi.org/10.1089/met.2010.0031.

53 L. Cusack et al., 'Blood type diets lack supporting evidence: a systematic review', *American Journal of Clinical Nutrition*, 98(1), July 2013, pp. 99–104, https://doi.org/10.3945/ajcn.113.058693.

54 J. Wang et al., 'ABO genotype, "blood-type" diet and cardiometabolic risk factors', *PLoS One*, 9(1), January 2014, e84749, https://doi.org/10.1371/journal.pone.0084749.

55 L. L. Hamm et al., 'Acid-Base Homeostasis', *Clinical Journal of the American Society of Nephrology*, 10(12), December 2015, pp. 2232–42, https://doi.org/10.2215/CJN.07400715.

56 T. R. Fenton and T. Huang, 'Systematic review of the association between dietary acid load, alkaline water and cancer', *BMJ Open*, 6(6), June 2016, e010438, https://doi.org/10.1136/bmjopen-2015-010438.

57 F. Gholami et al., 'Dietary Acid Load and Bone Health: A Systematic Review and Meta-Analysis of Observational Studies', *Frontiers in Nutrition*, May 2022, https://doi.org/10.3389/fnut.2022.869132.

58 D. N. Juurlink, 'Activated charcoal for acute overdose: a reappraisal', *British Journal of Clinical Pharmacology*, 81(3), March 2018, pp. 482–7, https://doi.org/10.1111/bcp.12793.

59 D. M. Grant, 'Detoxification pathways in the liver', *Journal of Inherited Metabolic Disease*, 14(4), 1991, pp. 421–30, https://doi.org/10.1007/BF01797915; X. X. Liu et al., 'Decreased skin-mediated detoxification contributes to oxidative stress and insulin resistance', *Experimental Diabetes Research*, 2012, e128694, https://doi.org/10.1155/2012/128694.

60 S. Kraljević Pavelić et al., 'Clinical Evaluation of a Defined Zeolite-Clinoptilolite Supplementation Effect on the Selected Blood Parameters of Patients', *Frontiers in Medicine* (Lausanne), 9, May 2022, e851782, https://doi.org/10.3389/fmed.2022.851782.

61 S. M. Phillips et al., 'Protein "requirements" beyond the RDA: implications for optimizing health', *Applied Physiology, Nutrition, and Metabolism*, 41(5), May 2016, pp. 565–72, https://doi.org/10.1139/apnm-2015-0550. Erratum in: *Applied Physiology, Nutrition, and Metabolism*, 47(5), May 2022, p. 615.

62 R. W. Morton et al., 'A systematic review, meta-analysis and meta-regression of the effect of protein supplementation on resistance training-induced gains in muscle mass and strength in healthy adults', *British Journal of Sports Medicine*, 52(6), March 2018, pp. 376–84, https://doi.org/10.1136/bjsports-2017-097608. Erratum in: *British Journal of Sports Medicine*, 54(19), October 2020, e7.

63 A. J. Hector and S. M. Phillips, 'Protein Recommendations for Weight Loss in Elite Athletes: A Focus on Body Composition and Performance', *International Journal of Sport Nutrition and Exercise Metabolism*, 28(2), March 2018, pp. 170–7, https://doi.org/10.1123/ijsnem.2017-0273.

64 B. J. Schoenfeld and A. A. Aragon, 'How much protein can the body use in a single meal for muscle-building? Implications for daily protein distribution', *Journal of the International Society of Sports Nutrition*, 15, 2018, https://doi.org/10.1186/s12970-018-0215-1.

65 B. C. Johnston et al., 'Comparison of weight loss among named diet programs in overweight and obese adults: a meta-analysis', *JAMA*, 312(9), September 2014, pp. 923–33, https://doi.org/10.1001/jama.2014.10397; L. Ge et al., 'Comparison of dietary macronutrient patterns of 14 popular named dietary programmes for weight and cardiovascular risk factor reduction in adults: systematic review and network meta-analysis of randomised trials', *BMJ*, April 2020, m696, https://doi.org/10.1136/bmj.m696.

Inflammation: From Fork to Flame

1 B. S. Rett and J. Whelan, 'Increasing dietary linoleic acid does not increase tissue arachidonic acid content in adults consuming Western-type diets: A systematic review', *Nutrition & Metabolism*, 10, June 2011, p. 36, https://doi.org/10.1186/1743-7075-8-36.

2 H. Tallima and R. El Ridi, 'Arachidonic acid: Physiological roles and potential health benefits – A review', *Journal of Advanced Research*, 11, November 2017, pp. 33–41, https://doi.org/10.1016/j.jare.2017.11.004.

3 J. K. Innes and P. C. Calder, 'Omega-6 fatty acids and inflammation', *Prostaglandins, Leukotrienes & Essential Fatty Acids*, 132, May 2018, pp. 41–8, https://doi.org/10.1016/j.plefa.2018.03.004.

4 S. M. Ajabnoor et al., 'Long-term effects of increasing omega-3, omega-6 and total polyunsaturated fats on inflammatory bowel disease and markers of inflammation: A systematic review and meta-analysis of randomized controlled trials', *European Journal of Nutrition*, 60(5), August 2021, pp. 2293–316, https://doi.org/10.1007/s00394-020-02413-y.

5 L. Schwingshackl et al., 'Effects of oils and solid fats on blood lipids: A systematic review and network meta-analysis', *Journal of Lipid Research*, 59(9), September 2018, pp. 1771–82, https://doi.org/10.1194/jlr.P085522.

6 V. H. Telle-Hansen et al., 'Does dietary fat affect inflammatory markers in overweight and obese individuals? – A review of randomized controlled trials from 2010 to 2016', *Genes & Nutrition*, 12, October 2017, p. 26, https://doi.org/10.1186/s12263-017-0580-4.

7 R. J. de Souza et al., 'Intake of saturated and trans unsaturated fatty acids and risk of all cause mortality, cardiovascular disease, and type 2 diabetes: Systematic review and meta-analysis of observational studies', *BMJ*, 351, August 2015, h3978, https://doi.org/10.1136/bmj.h3978.

8 S. Santos et al., 'Systematic review of saturated fatty acids on inflammation and circulating levels of adipokines', *Nutrition Research*, 33(9), September 2013, pp. 687–95, https://doi.org/10.1016/j.nutres.2013.07.002.

9 J. Praagman et al., 'Consumption of individual saturated fatty acids and the risk of myocardial infarction in a UK and a Danish cohort', *International Journal of Cardiology*, 279, March 2019, pp. 18–26, https://doi.org/10.1016/j.ijcard.2018.10.064.

10 R. Mensink, 'Effects of saturated fatty acids on serum lipids and lipoproteins: A systematic review and regression analysis', Geneva, World Health Organization, 2016.

11 R. T. Zijlstra, 'Binding Fatty Acids into Indigestible Calcium Soap: Removing a Piece of Pie', *Journal of Nutrition*, 151(5), May 2021, pp. 1053–4, https://doi.org/10.1093/jn/nxab045.

12 A. Bordoni et al., 'Dairy products and inflammation: A review of the clinical evidence', *Critical Reviews in Food Science and Nutrition*, 57(12), August 2017, pp. 2497–525, https://doi.org/10.1080/10408398.2014.967385.

13 S. P. Moosavian et al., 'Effects of dairy products consumption on inflammatory biomarkers among adults: A systematic review and meta-analysis of randomized controlled trials', *Nutrition, Metabolism & Cardiovascular Diseases*, 30(6), June 2020, pp. 872–88, https://doi.org/10.1016/j.numecd.2020.01.011.

14 Y. Kim and C. W. Park, 'Mechanisms of Adiponectin Action: Implication of Adiponectin Receptor Agonism in Diabetic Kidney Disease', *International Journal of Molecular Sciences*, 20(7), April 2019, p. 1782, https://doi.org/10.3390/ijms20071782.

15 C. Liang et al., 'Leucine Modulates Mitochondrial Biogenesis and SIRT1-AMPK Signaling in C2C12 Myotubes', *Journal of Nutrition and Metabolism*, 2014, 239750, https://doi.org/10.1155/2014/239750.

16 X. Zhang et al., 'Milk consumption and multiple health outcomes: Umbrella review of systematic reviews and meta-analyses in humans', *Nutrition & Metabolism*, 18(1), January 2021, p. 7, https://doi.org/10.1186/s12986-020-00527-y.

17 L. B. Sørensen et al., 'Effect of sucrose on inflammatory markers in overweight humans', *American Journal of Clinical Nutrition*, 82(2), August 2005, pp. 421–7, https://doi.org/10.1093/ajcn.82.2.421.

18 K. W. Della Corte et al., 'Effect of Dietary Sugar Intake on Biomarkers of Subclinical Inflammation: A Systematic Review and Meta-Analysis of Intervention Studies', *Nutrients*, 10(5), May 2018, p. 606, https://doi.org/10.3390/nu10050606.

19 G. Caio et al., 'Celiac disease: A comprehensive current review', *BMC Medicine*, 17(1), July 2019, p. 142, https://doi.org/10.1186/s12916-019-1380-z.

20 U. Volta et al., 'Study Group for Non-Celiac Gluten Sensitivity. An Italian prospective multicenter survey on patients suspected of having non-celiac gluten sensitivity', *BMC Medicine*, 12, May 2014, p. 85, https://doi.org/10.1186/1741-7015-12-85.

21 R. Krysiak et al., 'The Effect of Gluten-Free Diet on Thyroid Auto-immunity in Drug-Naïve Women with Hashimoto's Thyroiditis: A Pilot Study', *Experimental and Clinical Endocrinology & Diabetes*, 127(7), July 2019, pp. 417–22, https://doi.org/10.1055/a-0653-7108.

22 B. Niland and B. D. Cash, 'Health Benefits and Adverse Effects of a Gluten-Free Diet in Non-Celiac Disease Patients', *Gastroenterology & Hepatology*, 14(2), February 2018, pp. 82–91, https://pubmed.ncbi.nlm.nih.gov/29606920.

23 B. Lebwohl et al., 'Long term gluten consumption in adults without celiac disease and risk of coronary heart disease: prospective cohort study', *BMJ*, 357, May 2017, j1892, https://doi.org/10.1136/bmj.j1892.

24 B. Missbach et al., 'Gluten-free food database: the nutritional quality and cost of packaged gluten-free foods', *PeerJ*, October 2015, e1337, https://doi.org/10.7717/peerj.1337; A. Cardo et al., 'Nutritional Imbalances in Adult Celiac Patients Following a Gluten-Free Diet', *Nutrients*, 13(8), August 2021, p. 2877, https://doi.org/10.3390/nu13082877.

25 T. Suzuki, 'Regulation of the intestinal barrier by nutrients: The role of tight junctions', *Animal Science Journal*, 91(1), 2020, e13357, https://doi.org/10.1111/asj.13357.

26 P. H. Liu et al., 'Dietary Gluten Intake and Risk of Microscopic Col-itis Among US Women without Celiac Disease: A Prospective Cohort Study', *American Journal of Gastroenterology*, 114(1), January 2019, pp. 127–34, https://doi.org/10.1038/s41395-018-0267-5. Erratum in: *American Journal of Gastroenterology*, 114(5), May 2019, p. 837.

27 H. K. F. Henriques et al., 'Gluten-Free Diet Reduces Diet Quality and Increases Inflammatory Potential in Non-Celiac Healthy Women', *Journal of the American Nutrition Association*, 13, September 2021, pp. 1–9, https://doi.org/10.1080/07315724.2021.1962769.

28 J. Singh and K. Whelan, 'Limited availability and higher cost of glu-ten-free foods', *Journal of Human Nutrition and Dietetics*, 24(5), October 2011, pp. 479–86, https://doi.org/10.1111/j.1365-277X.2011.01160.x.

29 R. Pahwa et al., *Chronic Inflammation*, https://www.ncbi.nlm.nih.gov/books/NBK493173.

30 M. S. Ellulu et al., 'Obesity and inflammation: The linking mechanism and the complications', 13(4), *Archives of Medical Science*, June 2017, pp. 851–63, https://doi.org/10.5114/aoms.2016.58928.

31 R. Monteiro and I. Azevedo, 'Chronic inflammation in obesity and the metabolic syndrome', *Mediators of Inflammation*, 2010, e289645, https://doi.org/10.1155/2010/289645.

32 A. S. Greenstein et al., 'Local inflammation and hypoxia abolish the protective anticontractile properties of perivascular fat in obese patients', *Circulation*, 119(12), March 2009, pp. 1661–70, https://doi.org/10.1161/CIRCULATIONAHA.108.821181.

33 H. Kord Varkaneh et al., 'Dietary inflammatory index in relation to obesity and body mass index: A meta-analysis', *Nutrition & Food Science*, 48(5), 2018, pp. 702–21, https://doi.org/10.1108/NFS-09-2017-0203; M. A. Farhangi and M. Vajdi, 'The association between dietary inflammatory index and risk of central obesity in adults: An updated systematic review and meta-analysis', *International Journal for Vitamin and Nutrition Research*, 90(5–6), October 2020, pp. 535–52, https://doi.org/10.1024/0300-9831/a000648.

34 G. Talamonti et al., 'Aulus Cornelius Celsus and the Head Injuries', *World Neurosurgery*, 133, January 2020, pp. 127–34, https://doi.org/10.1016/j.wneu.2019.09.119.

35 P. M. Ridker et al., 'CANTOS Trial Group. Antiinflammatory Therapy with Canakinumab for Atherosclerotic Disease', *New England Journal of Medicine*, 377(12), September 2017, pp. 1119–31, https://doi.org/10.1056/NEJMoa1707914.

36 N. Shivappa et al., 'Designing and developing a literature-derived, population-based dietary inflammatory index', 17(8), *Public Health Nutrition*, August 2014, pp. 1689–96, https://doi.org/10.1017/S1368980013002115.

37 J. R. Hebert and L. J. Hofseth, *Diet Inflammation and Health*, Elsevier, 2022, p. 788.

38 R. Ginwala et al., 'Potential Role of Flavonoids in Treating Chronic Inflammatory Diseases with a Special Focus on the Anti-Inflammatory Activity of Apigenin', *Antioxidants* (Basel), 8(2), February 2019, p. 35, https://doi.org/10.3390/antiox8020035.

39 R. M. Uncles et al., 'Effects of red raspberry polyphenols and metabolites on the biomarkers of inflammation and insulin resistance in type 2 diabetes: A pilot study', *Food & Function*, 9, 2022, pp. 5166–76, https://doi.org/10.1039/D1FO02090K.

40 S. Kumar and A. K. Pandey, 'Chemistry and biological activities of flavonoids: An overview', *The Scientific World Journal*, December 2013, 162750, https://doi.org/10.1155/2013/162750.

41 A. Constantinou et al., 'Genistein inactivates bcl-2, delays the G2/M phase of the cell cycle, and induces apoptosis of human breast adenocarcinoma MCF-7 cells', *European Journal of Cancer*, 34(12), November 1998, pp. 1927–34, https://doi.org/10.1016/s0959-8049(98)00198-1.

42 A. Kaulmann and T. Bohn, 'Carotenoids, inflammation, and oxidative stress – implications of cellular signaling pathways and relation to chronic disease prevention', *Nutrition Research*, 34(11), November 2014, pp. 907–29, https://doi.org/10.1016/j.nutres.2014.07.010.

43 H. Zhou H et al., 'Saturated Fatty Acids in Obesity-Associated Inflammation', *Journal of Inflammation Research*, 13, January 2020, pp. 1–14, https://doi.org/10.2147/JIR.S229691.

44 C. J. Masson and R. P. Mensink, 'Exchanging saturated fatty acids for (n-6) polyunsaturated fatty acids in a mixed meal may decrease postprandial lipemia and markers of inflammation and endothelial activity in overweight men', *Journal of Nutrition*, 141(5), May 2011, pp. 816–21, https://doi.org/10.3945/jn.110.136432.

45 B. Sears and A. K. Saha, 'Dietary Control of Inflammation and Resolution', *Frontiers in Nutrition*, 8, August 2021, 709435, https://doi.org/10.3389/fnut.2021.709435.

46 J. Most et al., 'Calorie restriction in humans: An update', *Ageing Research Reviews*, 39, October 2017, pp. 36–45, https://doi.org/10.1016/j.arr.2016.08.005.

47 W. E. Kraus et al., '2 years of calorie restriction and cardiometabolic risk (CALERIE), exploratory outcomes of a multicentre, phase 2, randomised controlled trial', *Lancet Diabetes Endocrinology*, 7(9), September 2019, pp. 673–83, https://doi.org/10.1016/S2213-8587(19)30151-2.

48 P. Li et al., 'Amino acids and immune function', *British Journal of Nutrition*, 98(2), August 2007, pp. 237–52, https://doi.org/10.1017/S000711450769936X.

49 P. Newsholme, 'Cellular and metabolic mechanisms of nutrient actions in immune function', *European Journal of Clinical Nutrition*, September 2021, 75(9), pp. 1328–31, https://doi.org/10.1038/s41430-021-00960-z.

50 O. C. Witard et al., 'Protein Considerations for Optimising Skeletal Muscle Mass in Healthy Young and Older Adults', *Nutrients*, 8(4), March 2016, p. 181, https://doi.org/10.3390/nu8040181.

51 P. C. Calder, 'Omega-3 fatty acids and inflammatory processes', *Nutrients*, 2(3), March 2010, pp. 355–74, https://doi.org/10.3390/nu2030355.

52 J. K. Kiecolt-Glaser et al., 'Omega-3 supplementation lowers inflammation and anxiety in medical students: a randomized controlled trial', *Brain, Behavior, and Immunity*, 25(8), November 2011, pp. 1725–34, https://doi.org/10.1016/j.bbi.2011.07.229.

53 P. C. Calder, 'Omega-3 fatty acids and inflammatory processes: from molecules to man', *Biochemical Society Transactions*, 15;45(5), October 2017, pp. 1105–15, https://doi.org/10.1042/BST20160474.

54 K. Ganesan and B. Xu, 'Polyphenol-Rich Lentils and Their Health Promoting Effects', *International Journal of Molecular Sciences*, 18(11), November 2017, 10; p. 2390, https://doi.org/10.3390/ijms18112390.

55 L. S. McAnulty, et al., 'Effect of blueberry ingestion on natural killer cell counts, oxidative stress, and inflammation prior to and after 2.5 h of running', *Applied Physiology, Nutrition, and Metabolism*, December 2011, 36(6), pp. 976–84, https://doi.org/10.1139/h11-120.

Weight: The Big Fat Debate

1 '45% of people globally are currently trying to lose weight', Ipsos, 18 January 2021, https://www.ipsos.com/en/global-weight-and-actions.

2 A. E. Achari and S. K. Jain, 'Adiponectin, a Therapeutic Target for Obesity, Diabetes, and Endothelial Dysfunction', *International*

Journal of Molecular Sciences, 18(6), June 2017, p. 1321, https://doi.org/10.3390/ijms18061321.

3 C. D. Fryar et al., 'Prevalence of overweight, obesity, and severe obesity among adults aged 20 and over: United States, 1960–1962 through 2017–2018', NCHS Health E-Stats, Centers for Disease Control and Prevention, 2020, updated 8 February 2021 (accessed October 2022), www.cdc.gov/nchs/data/hestat/obesity-adult-17-18/obesity-adult.htm.

4 S. P. Messier et al., 'Weight loss reduces knee-joint loads in overweight and obese older adults with knee osteoarthritis', *Arthritis & Rheumatology*, 52(7), July 2005, pp. 2026–32, https://doi.org/10.1002/art.21139.

5 D. B. Sarwer and H. M. Polonsky, 'The Psychosocial Burden of Obesity', *Endocrinology and Metabolism Clinics of North America*, 45(3), September 2016, pp. 677–88, https://doi.org/10.1016/j.ecl.2016.04.016.

6 M. S. Kim et al., 'Association between adiposity and cardiovascular outcomes: an umbrella review and meta-analysis of observational and Mendelian randomization studies', *European Heart Journal*, 42(34), September 2021, pp. 3388–403, https://doi.org/10.1093/eurheartj/ehab454

7 A. Jayedi et al., 'Anthropometric and adiposity indicators and risk of type 2 diabetes: systematic review and dose-response meta-analysis of cohort studies', *BMJ*, 376, 2022, e067516, https://doi.org/10.1136/bmj-2021-067516.

8 M. Blagojevic et al., 'Risk factors for onset of osteoarthritis of the knee in older adults: A systematic review and meta-analysis', *Osteoarthritis and Cartilage*, 18(1), January 2010, pp. 24–33, https://doi.org/10.1016/j.joca.2009.08.010.

9 F. S. Luppino et al., 'Overweight, obesity, and depression: a systematic review and meta-analysis of longitudinal studies', *Archives of General Psychiatry*, 67(3), March 2010, pp. 220–9, https://doi.org/10.1001/archgenpsychiatry.2010.2.

10 M. Dobbins et al., 'The Association between Obesity and Cancer Risk: A Meta-Analysis of Observational Studies from 1985 to 2011', *ISRN Preventive Medicine*, April 2013, 680536, https://doi.org/10.5402/2013/680536.

11 A. Abdullah et al., 'The magnitude of association between overweight and obesity and the risk of diabetes: a meta-analysis of prospective cohort studies', *Diabetes Research and Clinical Practice*, 89(3), September 2010, pp. 309–19, https://doi.org/10.1016/j.diabres. 2010.04.012.

12 M. Dobbins et al. (2013).

13 G. Lippi and Mattiuzzi, 'Fried food and prostate cancer risk: Systematic review and meta-analysis', *International Journal of Food Sciences and Nutrition*, 66(5), 2015, pp. 587–9, https://doi.org/10.3109/0963748 6.2015.1056111.

14 M. Blüher, 'Metabolically Healthy Obesity', *Endocrine Reviews*, 41(3), May 2020, bnaa004, https://doi.org/10.1210/endrev/bnaa004.

15 F. Caleyachetty et al., 'Metabolically Healthy Obese and Incident Cardiovascular Disease Events Among 3.5 Million Men and Women', *Journal of the American College of Cardiology*, 70(12), September 2017, pp. 1429–37, https://doi.org/10.1016/j.jacc.2017.07.763.

16 R. Zheng et al., 'The long-term prognosis of cardiovascular disease and all-cause mortality for metabolically healthy obesity: A systematic review and meta-analysis', *Journal of Epidemiology and Community Health*, 70(10), October 2016, pp. 1024–31, https://doi.org/10.1136/jech-2015-206948; J. A. Bell et al., 'Metabolically healthy obesity and risk of incident type 2 diabetes: A meta-analysis of prospective cohort studies', *Obesity Reviews*, June 2014, 15(6), pp. 504–15, https://doi.org/10.1111/obr.12157.

17 E. A. Willis et al., 'Increased frequency of intentional weight loss associated with reduced mortality: a prospective cohort analysis', *BMC Medicine*, 18(1), September 2020, p. 248, https://doi.org/10.1186/s12916-020-01716-5.

18 J. Davis et al., 'Relationship of ethnicity and body mass index with the development of hypertension and hyperlipidemia', *Ethnicity & Disease*, 23(1), winter 2013, pp. 65–70, https://pubmed.ncbi.nlm.nih.gov/23495624/.

19 P. Misra et al., 'Relationship between body mass index and percentage of body fat, estimated by bio-electrical impedance among adult

females in a rural community of North India: A cross-sectional study', *Journal of Postgraduate Medicine*, 65(3), Summer 2019, pp. 134–140, https://doi.org/10.4103/jpgm.JPGM_218_18; M. O. Akindele et al., 'The Relationship Between Body Fat Percentage and Body Mass Index in Overweight and Obese Individuals in an Urban African Setting', *Journal of Public Health in Africa*, 7(1), August 2016, p. 515, https://doi.org/10.4081/jphia.2016.515.

20 C. Ranasinghe et al., 'Relationship between Body Mass Index (BMI) and body fat percentage, estimated by bioelectrical impedance, in a group of Sri Lankan adults: a cross sectional study', *BMC Public Health*, 13, September 2013, p. 797, https://doi.org/10.1186/1471-2458-13-797.

21 Y. Chen et al., 'Weight loss increases all-cause mortality in over-weight or obese patients with diabetes: A meta-analysis', *Medicine* (Baltimore), 97(35), August 2018, e12075, https://doi.org/10.1097/MD.0000000000012075; A. Huang et al., 'Association of magnitude of weight loss and weight variability with mortality and major cardiovascular events among individuals with type 2 diabetes mellitus A systematic review and meta-analysis', *Cardiovascular Diabetology*, 21, 2022, p. 78, https://doi.org/10.1186/s12933-022-01503-x.

22 A. N. Fabricatore et al., 'Intentional weight loss and changes in symptoms of depression: a systematic review and meta-analysis' *International Journal of Obesity*, 35(11), November 2011, pp. 1363–76 https://doi.org/10.1038/ijo.2011.2; S. B. Kritchevsky et al., 'Intentional weight loss and all-cause mortality: A meta-analysis of randomized clinical trials', *PLoS One*, 10(3), March 2015, e0121993 https://doi.org/10.1371/journal.pone.0121993.

23 R. S. Surwit et al., 'Metabolic and behavioral effects of a high-sucrose diet during weight loss', *American Journal of Clinical Nutrition*, 65(4) April 1997, pp. 908–15, https://doi.org/10.1093/ajcn/65.4.908.

24 Jane Fritsch, '95% regain lost weight, or do they?', *New York Times*, 25 May 1999, https://www.nytimes.com/1999/05/25/health/95-regain-lost-weight-or-do-they.html.

25 D. H. Ryan and S. R. Yockey, 'Weight Loss and Improvement in Comorbidity: Differences at 5%, 10%, 15%, and Over', *Current Obesity Reports*, 6(2), June 2017, pp. 187–94, https://doi.org/10.1007/s13679-017-0262-y.

26 J. W. Anderson et al., 'Long-term weight-loss maintenance: a meta-analysis of US studies', *American Journal of Clinical Nutrition*, November 2001, 74(5), pp. 579–84, https://doi.org/10.1093/ajcn/74.5.579.

27 M. M. Ibrahim, 'Subcutaneous and visceral adipose tissue: structural and functional differences', *Obesity Reviews*, 11(1), January 2010, pp. 11–8, https://doi.org/10.1111/j.1467-789X.2009.00623.x.

28 A. Jayedi et al., 'Central fatness and risk of all cause mortality: Systematic review and dose-response meta-analysis of 72 prospective cohort studies', *BMJ*, 370, September 2020, m3324, https://doi.org/10.1136/bmj.m3324.

29 R. J. Verheggen et al., 'A systematic review and meta-analysis on the effects of exercise training versus hypocaloric diet: Distinct effects on body weight and visceral adipose tissue', *Obesity Reviews*, 17(8), August 2016, pp. 664–90, https://doi.org/10.1111/obr.12406.

30 A. Bellicha et al., 'Effect of exercise training on weight loss, body composition changes, and weight maintenance in adults with overweight or obesity: An overview of 12 systematic reviews and 149 studies', *Obesity Reviews*, July 2021, 22(S4), e13256, https://doi.org/10.1111/obr.13256.

31 A. S. Wedell-Neergaard et al., 'Exercise-Induced Changes in Visceral Adipose Tissue Mass Are Regulated by IL-6 Signaling: A Randomized Controlled Trial', *Cell Metabolism*, 29(4), April 2019, pp. 844–55, e3, https://doi.org/10.1016/j.cmet.2018.12.007.

32 A. Tchernof and J. P. Després, 'Pathophysiology of human visceral obesity: An update', *Physiological Reviews*, 93(1), January 2013, pp. 359–404, https://doi.org/10.1152/physrev.00033.2011.

33 Y. H. Chang et al., 'Effect of exercise intervention dosage on reducing visceral adipose tissue: A systematic review and network meta-analysis of randomized controlled trials', *International Journal of Obesity* (London), 45(5), May 2021, pp. 982–97, https://doi.

org/10.1038/s41366-021-00767-9. Erratum in: *International Journal of Obesity*, 46(4), April 2022, p. 890.

34 A. M. Goss et al., 'Effects of diet macronutrient composition on body composition and fat distribution during weight maintenance and weight loss', *Obesity* (Silver Spring), 21(6), June 2013, pp. 1139–42. https://doi.org/10.1002/oby.20191.

35 P. K. Luukkonen et al., 'Saturated Fat Is More Metabolically Harmful for the Human Liver Than Unsaturated Fat or Simple Sugars', *Diabetes Care*, 41(8), August 2018, pp. 1732–9, https://doi.org/10.2337/dc18-0071.

36 K. Y. Park et al., 'Relationship between abdominal obesity and alcohol drinking pattern in normal-weight, middle-aged adults: The Korea National Health and Nutrition Examination Survey 2008-2013', *Public Health Nutrition*, 20(12), August 2017, pp. 2192–200. https://doi.org/10.1017/S1368980017001045; H. Schröder et al., 'Relationship of abdominal obesity with alcohol consumption at population scale', *European Journal of Nutrition*, 46(7), 2007, pp. 369–76. https://doi.org/10.1007/s00394-007-0674-7.

37 J. K. Kiecolt-Glaser et al., 'Daily stressors, past depression, and metabolic responses to high-fat meals: A novel path to obesity', *Biological Psychiatry*, 77(7), April 2015, pp. 653–60, https://doi.org/10.1016/j.biopsych.2014.05.018.

38 J. A. Swift et al., 'Weight bias among UK trainee dietitians, doctors, nurses and nutritionists', *Journal of Human Nutrition and Dietetics*, 26(4), August 2013, pp. 395–402, https://doi.org/10.1111/jhn.12019.

39 N. A. Schvey et al., 'The impact of weight stigma on caloric consumption', *Obesity* (Silver Spring), 19(10), October 2011, pp. 1957–62. https://doi.org/10.1038/oby.2011.204.

40 K. M. Lee et al., 'Weight stigma and health behaviors: evidence from the Eating in America Study', *International Journal of Obesity*, 45, 2021, 1499–1509, https://doi.org/10.1038/s41366-021-00814-5.

41 E. Karra et al., 'A link between FTO, ghrelin, and impaired brain food-cue responsivity', *Journal of Clinical Investigation*, August 2013, 123(8), pp. 3539–51, https://doi.org/10.1172/JCI44403. Epub 15 Jul 2015. PMID: 23867619; PMCID: PMC3726147.

42 A.J. Stunkard et al., 'The body-mass index of twins who have been reared apart', *New England Journal of Medicine*, 322(21), May 1990, pp. 1483–7, https://doi.org/10.1056/NEJM199005243222102.

43 S. M. Mason et al., 'Abuse victimization in childhood or adolescence and risk of food addiction in adult women', *Obesity* (Silver Spring), 21(12), December 2013, e775–81, https://doi.org/10.1002/oby.20500.

44 N. Parekh et al., 'Food insecurity among households with children during the COVID-19 pandemic: Results from a study among social media users across the United States', *Nutrition Journal*, 20, 2021, article 73, https://doi.org/10.1186/s12937-021-00732-2.

45 A. Tedstone et al., *Sugar reduction, achieving the 20%: A technical report outlining progress to date, guidelines for industry, 2015 baseline levels in key foods and next steps*, 2017, available from www.gov.uk/phe.

46 A. Elliott-Green et al., 'Sugar-sweetened beverages coverage in the British media: an analysis of public health advocacy versus pro-industry messaging', *BMJ Open*, 6(7), July 2016, e011295, https://doi.org/10.1136/bmjopen-2016-011295.

47 Action on Salt, 'Policy Position: UK Salt Reduction Strategy', https://www.actiononsalt.org.uk/media/action-on-salt/about/FINAL-Action-on-Salt-Policy-Brief.pdf.

48 S. Alonso et al., 'Impact of the 2003 to 2018 Population Salt Intake Reduction Program in England: A Modeling Study', *Hypertension*, 77(4), April 2021, pp. 1086–94, https://doi.org/10.1161/HYPERTENSIONAHA.120.16649.

Weight Loss: Achieving Sustainability

1 The National Weight Control Registry. Accessible at: http://www.nwcr.ws.

2 C. Leonie et al., 'Timing of daily calorie loading affects appetite and hunger responses without changes in energy metabolism in healthy subjects with obesity', *Cell Metabolism*, 34(10), 2022, pp. 1472–85, https://doi.org/10.1016/j.cmet.2022.08.001.

3 D. A. Raynor et al., 'Television viewing and long-term weight maintenance: Results from the National Weight Control Registry', *Obesity* (Silver Spring), 14(10), October 2006, pp. 1816–24, https://doi.org/10.1038/oby.2006.209.

4 Z. Alimoradi et al., 'Binge-Watching and Mental Health Problems: A Systematic Review and Meta-Analysis', *International Journal of Environmental Research and Public Health*, 19(15), August 2022, p. 9707, https://doi.org/10.3390/ijerph19159707.

5 A. Bellicha et al., 'Effect of exercise training on weight loss, body composition changes, and weight maintenance in adults with overweight or obesity: An overview of 12 systematic reviews and 149 studies', *Obesity Reviews*, 22(S4), July 2021, e13256, https://doi.org/10.1111/obr.13256.

6 K. R. Arlinghaus and C. A. Johnston, 'The Importance of Creating Habits and Routine', *American Journal of Lifestyle Medicine*, 13(2), December 2018, pp. 142–4, https://doi.org/10.1177/1559827618818044.

7 H. Pontzer et al., 'Constrained Total Energy Expenditure and Metabolic Adaptation to Physical Activity in Adult Humans', *Current Biology*, 26(3), February 2016, pp. 410–7, https://doi.org/10.1016/j.cub.2015.12.046.

8 C. K. Martin et al., 'Effect of different doses of supervised exercise on food intake, metabolism, and non-exercise physical activity: The E-MECHANIC randomized controlled trial', *American Journal of Clinical Nutrition*, 110(3), September 2019, pp. 583–92, https://doi.org/10.1093/ajcn/nqz054.

9 J. Westenhoefer et al., 'Behavioural correlates of successful weight reduction over 3 y. Results from the Lean Habits Study', *International Journal of Obesity and Related Metabolic Disorders*, 28(2), February 2004, pp. 334–5, https://doi.org/10.1038/sj.ijo.0802530.

10 A. Palascha et al., 'How does thinking in Black and White terms relate to eating behavior and weight regain?', *Journal of Health Psychology*, 20(5), May 2015, pp. 638–48, https://doi.org/10.1177/1359105315573440.

11 A. C. Berg et al., 'Flexible Eating Behavior Predicts Greater Weight Loss Following a Diet and Exercise Intervention in Older Women', *Journal of Nutrition in Gerontology and Geriatrics*, 37(1), 2018, pp. 14–29, https://doi.org/10.1080/21551197.2018.1435433.

12 V. Loria-Kohen et al., 'Evaluation of the usefulness of a low-calorie diet with or without bread in the treatment of overweight/obesity', *Clinical Nutrition*, 31(4), August 2012, pp. 455–61, https://doi.org/10.1016/j.clnu.2011.12.002.

13 P. Srikanthan and A. S. Karlamangla, 'Muscle mass index as a predictor of longevity in older adults', *American Journal of Medicine*, 127(6), June 2014, pp. 547–53, https://doi.org/10.1016/j.amjmed.2014.02.007.

14 S. K. Gebauer et al., 'Food processing and structure impact the metabolizable energy of almonds', *Food & Function*, 7(10), October 2016, pp. 4231–8, https://doi.org/10.1039/c6fo01076h.

15 S. E. Berry et al., 'Manipulation of lipid bioaccessibility of almond seeds influences postprandial lipemia in healthy human subjects', *American Journal of Clinical Nutrition*, 88(4), October 2008, pp. 922–9, https://doi.org/10.1093/ajcn/88.4.922.

16 B. Dioneda et al., 'A Gluten-Free Meal Produces a Lower Postprandial Thermogenic Response Compared to an Iso-Energetic/Macronutrient Whole Food or Processed Food Meal in Young Women: A Single-Blind Randomized Cross-Over Trial', *Nutrients*, 12(7), July 2020, p. 2035, https://doi.org/10.3390/nu12072035.

17 S. B. Barr and J. C. Wright, 'Postprandial energy expenditure in whole-food and processed-food meals: Implications for daily energy expenditure', *Food Nutrition Research*, July 2010, p. 54, https://doi.org/10.3402/fnr.v54i0.5144.

18 M. Abbasalizad et al., 'Sugar-sweetened beverages intake and the risk of obesity in children: An updated systematic review and dose-response meta-analysis', *Pediatric Obesity*, 17(8), August 2022, e12914, https://doi.org/10.1111/ijpo.12914.

19 K. D. Hall et al., 'Ultra-Processed Diets Cause Excess Calorie Intake and Weight Gain: An Inpatient Randomized Controlled Trial of Ad Libitum Food Intake', *Cell Metabolism*, 30(1), July 2019, pp. 67–77, e3,

https://doi.org/10.1016/j.cmet.2019.05.008. Erratum in: *Cell Metabolism*, 32(4), October 2020, p. 690.

20 R. E. Brown et al., 'Calorie Estimation in Adults Differing in Body Weight Class and Weight Loss Status', *Medicine & Science in Sports & Exercise*, 48(3), March 2016, pp. 521–6, https://doi.org/10.1249/MSS.0000000000000796.

21 C. M. Champagne et al., 'Energy intake and energy expenditure: A controlled study comparing dietitians and non-dietitians', *Journal of the American Dietetic Association*, 102(10), October 2002, pp. 1428–32, https://doi.org/10.1016/s0002-8223(02)90316-0.

22 C. C. Simpson and S. E. Mazzeo, 'Calorie counting and fitness tracking technology: Associations with eating disorder symptomatology', *Eating Behaviors*, 26, August 2017, pp. 89–92, https://doi.org/10.1016/j.eatbeh.2017.02.002.

23 J. Linardon and M. Messer, 'My Fitness Pal usage in men: Associations with eating disorder symptoms and psychosocial impairment', *Eating Behaviors*, 33, April 2019, pp. 13–17, https://doi.org/10.1016/j.eatbeh.2019.02.003.

24 G. Cowburn and L. Stockley, 'Consumer understanding and use of nutrition labelling: a systematic review', *Public Health Nutrition*, 8(1), February 2005, pp. 21–8, https://doi.org/10.1079/phn2005666.

25 R. Jumpertz et al., 'Food label accuracy of common snack foods', *Obesity* (Silver Spring), 21(1), January 2013, pp. 164–9, https://doi.org/10.1002/oby.20185.

26 L. E. Urban et al., 'The accuracy of stated energy contents of reduced-energy, commercially prepared foods', *Journal of the American Dietetic Association*, 110(1), January 2010, pp. 116–23, https://doi.org/10.1016/j.jada.2009.10.003.

27 N. D. McGlynn et al., 'Low- and No-Calorie Sweetened Beverages as a Replacement for Sugar-Sweetened Beverages with Body Weight and Cardiometabolic Risk: A Systematic Review and Meta-analysis', *JAMA Network Open*, 5(3), March 2022, e222092, https://doi.org/10.1001/jamanetworkopen.2022.2092.

28 E. Robinson et al., 'A systematic review and meta-analysis examining the effect of eating rate on energy intake and hunger', *American Journal of Clinical Nutrition*, 100(1), July 2014, pp. 123–51, https://doi.org/10.3945/ajcn.113.081745.

29 B. Wansink et al., 'Ice cream illusions bowls, spoons, and self-served portion sizes', *American Journal of Preventive Medicine*, 31(3), September 2006, pp. 240–3, https://doi.org/10.1016/j.amepre.2006.04.003.

30 L. J. James et al., 'Eating with a smaller spoon decreases bite size, eating rate and ad libitum food intake in healthy young males', *British Journal of Nutrition*, 120(7), October 2018, pp. 830–7, https://doi.org/10.1017/S0007114518002246.

Chrononutrition and Sleep: Time on Your Plate

1 G. Asher and P. Sassone-Corsi, 'Time for food: The intimate interplay between nutrition, metabolism, and the circadian clock', *Cell*, 161(1), March 2015, pp. 84–92, https://doi.org/10.1016/j.cell.2015.03.015.

2 A. M. Haase et al., 'Gastrointestinal motility during sleep assessed by tracking of telemetric capsules combined with polysomnography – a pilot study', *Clinical and Experimental Gastroenterology*, 8, December 2015, pp. 327–32, https://doi.org/10.2147/CEG.S91964

3 S. Almoosawi et al., 'Daily profiles of energy and nutrient intakes: Are eating profiles changing over time?', *European Journal of Clinical Nutrition*, 66(6), June 2012, pp. 678–86, https://doi.org/10.1038/ejcn.2011.210.

4 C. Gu et al., 'Metabolic Effects of Late Dinner in Healthy Volunteers – A Randomized Crossover Clinical Trial', *Journal of Clinical Endocrinology and Metabolism*, 105(8), August 2020, pp. 2789–802, https://doi.org/10.1210/clinem/dgaa354.

5 M. Hibi et al., 'Nighttime snacking reduces whole body fat oxidation and increases LDL cholesterol in healthy young women', *American Journal of Physiology-Regulatory, Integrative and Comparative*

Physiology, 304(2), January 2013, R94–R101, https://doi.org/10.1152/ajpregu.00115.2012.

6 L. K. Cella et al., 'Diurnal rhythmicity of human cholesterol synthesis: Normal pattern and adaptation to simulated "jet lag"', *American Physiological Society*, 269(3 Pt 1), September 1995, e489–98, https://doi.org/10.1152/ajpendo.1995.269.3.E489.

7 Brian A. Ference et al., 'Low-density lipoproteins cause atherosclerotic cardiovascular disease. 1. Evidence from genetic, epidemiologic, and clinical studies. A consensus statement from the European Atherosclerosis Society Consensus Panel', *European Heart Journal*, 38(32), August 2017, pp. 2459–72, https://doi.org.UK/10.1093/eurheartj/ehx144; E. P. Navarese et al., 'Association Between Baseline LDL-C Level and Total and Cardiovascular Mortality After LDL-C Lowering: A Systematic Review and Meta-analysis', *JAMA*, 319(15), April 2018, pp. 1566–79, https://doi.org/10.1001/jama.2018.2525. Erratum in: *JAMA*, 320(13), October 2018, p. 1387.

8 G. K. W. Leung et al., 'Time of day difference in postprandial glucose and insulin responses: Systematic review and meta-analysis of acute postprandial studies', *Chronobiology International*, 37(3), March 2020, pp. 311–26, https://doi.org/10.1080/07420528.2019.1683856.

9 Y. Altuntaş, 'Postprandial Reactive Hypoglycemia', *Sisli Etfal Hastan Tip Bulteni*, 53(3), August 2019, pp. 215–20, https://doi.org/10.14744 SEMB.2019.59455.

10 K. R. Westerterp, 'Diet induced thermogenesis', *Nutrition & Metab olism*, 1(1), August 2004, p. 5, https://doi.org/10.1186/1743-7075-1-5.

11 C. J. Morris et al., 'The Human Circadian System Has a Dominatin Role in Causing the Morning/Evening Difference in Diet-Induce Thermogenesis', *Obesity* (Silver Spring), 23(10), October 2015, p 2053–8, https://doi.org/10.1002/oby.21189; S. Bo et al., 'Is the timin of caloric intake associated with variation in diet-induced therm genesis and in the metabolic pattern? A randomized cross-ove study', *International Journal of Obesity* (London), 39(12), Decembe 2015, pp. 1689–95, https://doi.org/10.1038/ijo.2015.138.

12 L. Ruddick-Collins et al., 'Circadian Rhythms in Resting Metabolic Rate Account for Apparent Daily Rhythms in the Thermic Effect of Food', *Journal of Clinical Endocrinology and Metabolism*, 107(2), January 2022, e708–e715, https://doi.org/10.1210/clinem/dgab654.

13 M. H. Alhussain et al., 'Impact of isoenergetic intake of irregular meal patterns on thermogenesis, glucose metabolism, and appetite: a randomized controlled trial', *American Journal of Clinical Nutrition*, 115(1), January 2022, pp. 284–97; M. H. Alhussain et al., 'Irregular meal-pattern effects on energy expenditure, metabolism, and appetite regulation: A randomized controlled trial in healthy normal-weight women', *American Journal of Clinical Nutrition*, 104(1), July 2016, pp. 21–32, https://doi.org/10.3945/ajcn.115.125401.

14 T. P. Aird et al., 'Effects of fasted vs fed-state exercise on performance and post-exercise metabolism: A systematic review and meta-analysis', *Scandinavian Journal of Medicine & Science in Sports*, 28(5), May 2018, pp. 1476–93, https://doi.org/10.1111/sms.13054.

15 M. P. St-Onge et al., 'Effects of Diet on Sleep Quality', *Advances in Nutrition*, 7(5), September 2016, pp. 938–49, https://doi.org/10.3945/an.116.012336.

16 H. S. Dashti et al., 'Late eating is associated with cardiometabolic risk traits, obesogenic behaviors, and impaired weight loss', *American Journal of Clinical Nutrition*, 113(1), October 2020, pp. 154–61, https://doi.org/10.1093/ajcn/nqaa264; J. Lopez-Minguez et al., 'Timing of Breakfast, Lunch, and Dinner. Effects on Obesity and Metabolic Risk', *Nutrients*, November 2019, 1(11), p. 2624, https://doi.org/10.3390/nu11112624.

17 A. Madjd et al., 'Effects of consuming later evening meal v. earlier evening meal on weight loss during a weight loss diet: a randomised clinical trial', *British Journal of Nutrition*, 126(4), August 2021, pp. 632–40, https://doi.org/10.1017/S0007114520004456.

18 D. Jakubowicz et al., 'High caloric intake at breakfast vs. dinner differentially influences weight loss of overweight and obese women', *Obesity* (Silver Spring), 21(12), December 2013, pp. 2504–12, https://doi.org/10.1002/oby.20460.

19 M. Lombardo et al., 'Morning meal more efficient for fat loss in a 3-month lifestyle intervention', *Journal of the American Nutrition Association*, 33(3), 2014, pp. 198–205, https://doi.org/10.1080/07315724.2013.863169.

20 L. Ruddick-Collins et al., 'Timing of daily calorie loading affects appetite and hunger responses without changes in energy metabolism in healthy subjects with obesity', *Cell Metabolism*, 34(10), October 2022, pp. 1472–85, https://doi.org/10.1016/j.cmet.2022.08.001.

21 K. Sievert et al., 'Effect of breakfast on weight and energy intake: systematic review and meta-analysis of randomised controlled trials', *BMJ*, 364, January 2019, p. 142, https://doi.org/10.1136/bmj.l42.

22 S. Sharma and M. Kavuru, 'Sleep and metabolism: An overview', *International Journal of Endocrinology*, 2010, e270832, https://www.doi.org/10.1155/2010/270832.

23 K. D. Kochanek et al., 'Mortality in the United States, 2013', *NCHS Data Brief*, 178, December 2014, pp. 1–8.

24 M. H. Yazdanpanah et al., 'Short sleep is associated with higher prevalence and increased predicted risk of cardiovascular diseases in an Iranian population: Fasa PERSIAN Cohort Study', *Scientific Reports*, 10(1), March 2020, p. 4608, https://doi.org/10.1038/s41598-020-61506-0.

25 M. R. Irwin et al., 'Sleep Disturbance, Sleep Duration, and Inflammation: A Systematic Review and Meta-Analysis of Cohort Studies and Experimental Sleep Deprivation', *Biology Psychiatry*, 80(1), July 2016, pp. 40–52, https://doi.org/10.1016/j.biopsych.2015.05.014.

26 V. Kothari et al., 'Sleep interventions and glucose metabolism: systematic review and meta-analysis', *Sleep Medicine*, 78, February 2021, pp. 24–35, https://doi.org/10.1016/j.sleep.2020.11.035.

27 K. Lo et al., 'Subjective sleep quality, blood pressure, and hypertension: a meta-analysis', *Journal of Clinical Hypertension* (Greenwich), 20(3), March 2018, pp. 592–605, https://doi.org/10.1111/jch.13220.

28 J. L. Broussard et al., 'Impaired insulin signaling in human adipocytes after experimental sleep restriction: A randomized, crossover study', *Annals of Internal Medicine*, 157(8), October 2012, pp. 549–, https://doi.org/10.7326/0003-4819-157-8-201210160-00005.

29 Lee D. Y. et al., 'Sleep duration and the risk of type 2 diabetes: A community-based cohort study with a 16-year follow-up', *Endocrinology and Metabolism*, 38(1), February 2023, pp. 146–55, https://pubmed.ncbi.nlm.nih.gov/36740966.

30 F. P. Cappuccio et al., 'Meta-analysis of short sleep duration and obesity in children and adults', *Sleep*, 31(5), May 2008, pp. 619–26, https://doi.org/10.1093/sleep/31.5.619.

31 K. Spiegel et al., 'Brief communication: Sleep curtailment in healthy young men is associated with decreased leptin levels, elevated ghrelin levels, and increased hunger and appetite', *Annals of Internal Medicine*, 141(11), December 2004, pp. 846–50, https://doi.org/10.7326/0003-4819-11-200412070-00008.

32 C. Chin-Chance et al., 'Twenty-four-hour leptin levels respond to cumulative short-term energy imbalance and predict subsequent intake', *Journal of Clinical Endocrinology and Metabolism*, 85(8), August 2000, pp. 2685–91, https://doi.org.uk/10.1210/jcem.85.8.6755; S. Taheri et al., 'Short sleep duration is associated with reduced leptin, elevated ghrelin, and increased body mass index', *PLoS Med*, 1(3), December 2004, e62, https://doi.org/10.1371/journal.pmed.0010062.

33 A. Guyon et al., 'Adverse effects of two nights of sleep restriction on the hypothalamic–pituitary–adrenal axis in healthy men', *Journal of Clinical Endocrinology and Metabolism*, 99, 2014, pp. 2861–8, https://doi.org/10.1210/jc.2013-4254; R. Leproult et al., 'Sleep loss results in an elevation of cortisol levels the next evening', *Sleep*, 20, 1997, pp. 865–70, https://pubmed.ncbi.nlm.nih.gov/9415946.

34 A. M. Chao et al., 'Stress, cortisol, and other appetite-related hormones: Prospective prediction of 6-month changes in food cravings and weight', *Obesity* (Silver Spring), 25(4), 2017, pp. 713–20, https://doi.org/10.1002/oby.21790.

35 H. K. Al Khatib et al., 'The effects of partial sleep deprivation on energy balance: a systematic review and meta-analysis', *European Journal of Clinical Nutrition*, 71(5), May 2017, pp. 614–24, https://doi.org/10.1038/ejcn.2016.201. The analysis mentioned in the footnote

is: B. Zhu, 'Effects of sleep restriction on metabolism-related parameters in healthy adults: A comprehensive review and meta-analysis of randomized controlled trials', *Sleep Medicine Reviews*, 45, 2019, pp. 18–30, https://doi.org/10.1016/j.smrv.2019.02.002.

36 B. A. Dolezal et al., 'Interrelationship between Sleep and Exercise: A Systematic Review', *Advances in Preventive Medicine*, 2017, 1364387, https://doi.org/10.1155/2017/1364387.

37 S. I. Iao et al., 'Associations between bedtime eating or drinking, sleep duration and wake after sleep onset: Findings from the American time use survey', *British Journal of Nutrition*, 13, September 2021, pp. 1–10, https://doi.org.10.1017/S0007114521003597; N. Chung et al., 'Does the Proximity of Meals to Bedtime Influence the Sleep of Young Adults? A Cross-Sectional Survey of University Students', *International Journal of Environmental Research and Public Health*, 17(8), 2020, p. 2677, https://doi.org/10.1155/2017/1364387.

The Gut Microbiome: Man's Best Friend(s)

1 J. Lederberg, 'Infectious history', *Science*, 288(5464), April 2000, pp. 287–93, https://doi.org/10.1126/science.288.5464.287.

2 E. R. Leeming et al., 'Effect of Diet on the Gut Microbiota: Rethinking Intervention Duration', *Nutrients*, 11(12), November 2019, p. 2862, https://doi.org/10.3390/nu11122862.

3 K. AlFaleh and J. Anabrees, 'Probiotics for prevention of necrotizing enterocolitis in preterm infants', *Cochrane Database of Systematic Reviews*, 4, April 2014, CD005496, https://doi.org/10.1002/14651858. CD005496.pub4.

4 L. Satish Kumar et al., 'Probiotics in Irritable Bowel Syndrome: A Review of Their Therapeutic Role', *Cureus*, 14(4), 2022, e24240, https://doi.org/10.7759/cureus.24240.

5 S. Guglielmetti et al., 'Randomised clinical trial: *Bifidobacterium bifidum* MIMBb75 significantly alleviates irritable bowel syndrome and improves quality of life – a double-blind, placebo-controlled study'

Notes

Alimentary Pharmacology & Therapeutics, May 2011, 33(10), pp. 1123–32, https://doi.org/10.1111/j.1365-2036.2011.04633.x.

6 N. B. Kristensen et al., 'Alterations in fecal microbiota composition by probiotic supplementation in healthy adults: a systematic review of randomized controlled trials', *Genome Medicine*, 8(1), May 2016, article 52, https://doi.org/10.1186/s13073-016-0300-5.

7 J. Alvar et al., 'Implications of asymptomatic infection for the natural history of selected parasitic tropical diseases', *Seminars in Immunopathology*, 42(3), June 2020, pp. 231–46, https://doi.org/10.1007/s00281-020-00796-y.

8 H. Kiani et al., 'Prevalence, risk factors and symptoms associated to intestinal parasite infections among patients with gastrointestinal disorders in Nahavand, Western Iran', *Journal of the Institute of Tropical Medicine of São Paulo*, 58, 2016, p. 42, https://doi.org/10.1590/S1678-9946201658042.

9 J. Gocki and Z. Bartuzi, 'Role of immunoglobulin G antibodies in diagnosis of food allergy', *Advances in Dermatology and Allergology*, 33(4), August 2016, pp. 253–6, https://doi.org/10.5114/ada.2016.61600.

10 F. J. Ruiz-Ojeda et al., 'Effects of Sweeteners on the Gut Microbiota: A Review of Experimental Studies and Clinical Trials', *Advances in Nutrition*, 10, January 2019, S31–S48, https://doi.org/10.1093/advances/nmy037.

11 A. R. Lobach et al., 'Assessing the *in vivo* data on low/no-calorie sweeteners and the gut microbiota', *Food and Chemical Toxicology*, 124, February 2019, pp. 385–99, https://doi.org/10.1016/j.fct.2018.12.005.

2 N. D. McGlynn et al., 'Association of Low- and No-Calorie Sweetened Beverages as a Replacement for Sugar-Sweetened Beverages with Body Weight and Cardiometabolic Risk: A Systematic Review and Meta-analysis', *JAMA Network Open*, 5(3), March 2022, e222092, https://doi.org/10.1001/jamanetworkopen.2022.2092; S. Pavanello et al., 'Non-sugar sweeteners and cancer: Toxicological and epidemiological evidence', *Regulatory Toxicology and Pharmacology*, 139, March 2023, 105369, https://doi.org/10.1016/j.yrtph.2023.105369.

13 E. C. Gritz and V. Bhandari, 'The human neonatal gut microbiome: A brief review', *Frontiers in Pediatrics*, 3, March 2015, p. 17, https://doi.org/10.3389/fped.2015.00017. Erratum in: ibid., p. 60.

14 M. G. Dominguez-Bello et al., 'Delivery mode shapes the acquisition and structure of the initial microbiota across multiple body habitats in newborns', *Proceedings of the National Academy of Sciences of the United States of America*, 107(26), June 2010, pp. 11971–5, https://doi.org/10.1073/pnas.1002601107.

15 J. Neu and J. Rushing, 'Cesarean versus vaginal delivery: Long-term infant outcomes and the hygiene hypothesis', *Clinics in Perinatology*, 38(2), June 2011, pp. 321–31, https://doi.org/10.1016/j.clp.2011.03.008.

16 H. Okada et al. (2010).

17 A. O'Sullivan et al., 'The Influence of Early Infant-Feeding Practices on the Intestinal Microbiome and Body Composition in Infants', *Nutrition and Metabolic Insights*, December 2015, 8(Suppl 1), pp. 1–9, https://doi.org/10.4137/NMI.S29530. Erratum in: *Nutrition and Metabolic Insights*, (Suppl 1) October 2016, p. 87.

18 M. Wiciński et al., 'Human Milk Oligosaccharides: Health Benefits, Potential Applications in Infant Formulas, and Pharmacology', *Nutrients*, 12(1), January 2020, p. 266, https://doi.org/10.3390/nu12010266.

19 G. K. John and G. E. Mullin, 'The Gut Microbiome and Obesity', *Current Oncology Reports*, 18(7), July 2016, p. 45, https://doi.org/10.1007/s11912-016-0528-7; R. E. Ley et al., 'Microbial ecology: human gut microbes associated with obesity', *Nature*, 444(7122), December 2006, pp. 1022–3, https://doi.org/10.1038/4441022a.

20 P. Ojeda et al., 'Nutritional modulation of gut microbiota – the impact on metabolic disease pathophysiology', *Journal of Nutritional Biochemistry*, 28, February 2016, pp. 191–200, https://doi.org/10.1016/j.jnutbio.2015.08.013.

21 A. C. Gomes et al., 'The human gut microbiota: Metabolism and perspective in obesity', *Gut Microbes*, 9(4), July 2018, pp. 308–25, https://doi.org/10.1080/19490976.2018.1465157.

22 R. Liu et al., 'Gut microbiome and serum metabolome alterations in obesity and after weight-loss intervention', *Nature Medicine*, 23(7), July 2017, pp. 859–68, https://doi.org/10.1038/nm.4358.

23 P. J. Turnbaugh et al., 'An obesity-associated gut microbiome with increased capacity for energy harvest', *Nature*, 444(7122), December 2006, pp. 1027–31, https://doi.org/10.1038/nature05414.

24 C. Sanmiguel et al., 'Gut Microbiome and Obesity: A Plausible Explanation for Obesity', *Current Obesity Reports*, 4(2), June 2015, pp. 250–61, https://doi.org/10.1007/s13679-015-0152-0.

25 M. M. Finucane et al., 'A taxonomic signature of obesity in the microbiome? Getting to the guts of the matter', *PLoS One*, 9(1), January 2014, e84689, https://doi.org/10.1371/journal.pone.0084689.

26 A. E. Morgan et al., 'Cholesterol metabolism: A review of how ageing disrupts the biological mechanisms responsible for its regulation', *Ageing Research Reviews*, 27, May 2016, pp. 108–24, https://doi.org/10.1016/j.arr.2016.03.008.

27 A. Grefhorst et al., 'The TICE Pathway: Mechanisms and Lipid-Lowering Therapies', *Methodist Debakey Cardiovascular Journal*, 15(1), January 2019, pp. 70–6, https://doi.org/10.14797/mdcj-15-1-70.

28 J. Fu et al., 'The Gut Microbiome Contributes to a Substantial Proportion of the Variation in Blood Lipids', *Circulation Research*, 117(9), October 2015, pp. 817–24, https://doi.org/10.1161/CIRCRESAHA.115.306807.

29 J. M. Lattimer and H. D. Haub, 'Effects of dietary fiber and its components on metabolic health', *Nutrients*, 2(12), December 2010, pp. 1266–89, https://doi.org/10.3390/nu2121266.

30 L. Scalfi et al., 'Effect of dietary fiber on postprandial thermogenesis', *International Journal of Obesity*, 11(Suppl 1), 1987, pp. 95–9, https://pubmed.ncbi.nlm.nih.gov/3032832.

31 A. N. Reynolds et al., 'Dietary fiber in hypertension and cardiovascular disease management: Systematic review and meta-analyses', *BMC Medicine*, 20(1), April 2022, p. 139, https://doi.org/10.1186/s12916-022-02328-x; D. E. Threapleton et al., 'Dietary fiber intake

and risk of cardiovascular disease: systematic review and meta-analysis', *BMJ*, 347, 2013, https://doi.org/10.1136/bmj.f6879.

32 I. Miller, 'The gut–brain axis: Historical reflections', *Microbial Ecology in Health and Disease*, 29(1), November 2018, 1542921, https://doi.org/10.1080/16512235.2018.1542921.

33 T. Alexander et al., 'Effect of three antibacterial drugs in lowering blood & stool ammonia production in hepatic encephalopathy', *Indian Journal of Medical Research*, 96, October 1992, pp. 292–6, https://pubmed.ncbi.nlm.nih.gov/1459672/.

34 P. Bercik et al., 'The intestinal microbiota affect central levels of brain-derived neurotropic factor and behavior in mice', *Gastroenterology*, 141(2), August 2011, pp. 599–609, https://doi.org/10.1053/j.gastro.2011.04.052.

35 M. Messaoudi et al., 'Assessment of psychotropic-like properties of a probiotic formulation (*Lactobacillus helveticus* R0052 and *Bifidobacterium* longum R0175) in rats and human subjects', *British Journal of Nutrition*, March 2011, 105(5), pp. 755–64, https://doi.org/10.1017/S0007114510004319.

36 B. Müller et al., 'Fecal Short-Chain Fatty Acid Ratios as Related to Gastrointestinal and Depressive Symptoms in Young Adults', *Psychosomatic Medicine*, 83(7), September 2021, pp. 693–9, https://doi.org/10.1097/PSY.0000000000000965.

37 G. Clarke et al., 'A Distinct Profile of Tryptophan Metabolism along the Kynurenine Pathway Downstream of Toll-Like Receptor Activation in Irritable Bowel Syndrome', *Frontiers in Pharmacology*, 3 May 2012, p. 90, https://doi.org/10.3389/fphar.2012.00090.

38 H. M. Parracho et al., 'Differences between the gut microflora of children with autistic spectrum disorders and that of healthy children', *Journal of Medical Microbiology*, 54 (Pt 10), October 2005, pp. 987–91, https://doi.org/10.1099/jmm.0.46101-0; S. J. Chen et al. 'Association of Fecal and Plasma Levels of Short-Chain Fatty Acid with Gut Microbiota and Clinical Severity in Patients with Parkinson Disease', *Neurology*, 98(8), February 2022, e848–e858, https://doi.org/10.1212/WNL.0000000000013225.

39 K. Tillisch et al., 'Consumption of fermented milk product with probiotic modulates brain activity', *Gastroenterology*, 144(7), June 2013, pp. 1394–401, https://doi.org/10.1053/j.gastro.2013.02.043; Messaoudi et al. (2011).

40 L. A. David et al., 'Diet rapidly and reproducibly alters the human gut microbiome', *Nature*, 505(7484), 23 January 2014, pp. 559–63, https://doi.org/10.1038/nature12820.

41 H. L. Simpson and B. J. Campbell, 'Review article: Dietary fiber-microbiota interactions', *Alimentary Pharmacology & Therapeutics*, 42(2), July 2015, pp. 158–79, https://doi.org/10.1111/apt.13248.

42 S. Devkota and E. B. Chang, 'Interactions between Diet, Bile Acid Metabolism, Gut Microbiota, and Inflammatory Bowel Diseases', *Digestive Diseases*, 33(3), 2015, pp. 351–6, https://doi.org/10.1159/000371687.

43 S. M. Ajabnoor et al., 'Long-term effects of increasing omega-3, omega-6 and total polyunsaturated fats on inflammatory bowel disease and markers of inflammation: A systematic review and meta-analysis of randomized controlled trials', *European Journal of Nutrition*, 60(5), August 2021, pp. 2293–316, https://doi.org/10.1007/s00394-020-02413-y.

44 A. N. Ananthakrishnan et al., 'Association between reduced plasma 25-hydroxy vitamin D and increased risk of cancer in patients with inflammatory bowel diseases', *Clinical Gastroenterology and Hepatology*, 12(5), May 2014, pp. 821–7, https://doi.org/10.1016/j.cgh.2013.10.011.

45 N. Narula et al., 'Impact of High-Dose Vitamin D3 Supplementation in Patients with Crohn's Disease in Remission: A Pilot Randomized Double-Blind Controlled Study', *Digestive Diseases and Sciences*, 62(2), February 2017, pp. 448–55, https://doi.org/10.1007/s10620-016-4396-7.

46 A. Clark and N. Mach, 'Role of Vitamin D in the Hygiene Hypothesis: The Interplay between Vitamin D, Vitamin D Receptors, Gut Microbiota, and Immune Response', *Frontiers in Immunology*, 7, December 2016, p. 627, https://doi.org/10.3389/fimmu.2016.00627.

47 C. S. Brotherton et al., 'Avoidance of Fiber Is Associated with Greate Risk of Crohn's Disease Flare in a 6-Month Period', *Clinical Gastro enterology and Hepatology*, 14(8), August 2016, pp. 1130–6, https://doi org/10.1016/j.cgh.2015.12.029; A. Pituch-Zdanowska et al., 'The role o dietary fibre in inflammatory bowel disease', *Przeglad Gastroenterolog iczny* 2015, 10(3), pp. 135–41, https://doi.org/10.5114/pg.2015.52753.

48 X. Liu et al., 'Dietary fibre intake reduces risk of inflammatory bowe disease: Result from a meta-analysis', *Nutrition Research*, 35(9), Septem ber 2015, pp. 753–8, https://doi.org/10.1016/j.nutres.2015.05.021.

49 H. C. Wastyk et al., 'Gut-microbiota-targeted diets modulate humai immune status', *Cell*, 184(16), August 2021, pp. 4137–53, https://do org/10.1016/j.cell.2021.06.019.

50 L. Saha, 'Irritable bowel syndrome: Pathogenesis, diagnosis treatment, and evidence-based medicine', *World Journal of Gastre enterology*, 20(22), June 2014, pp. 6759–73, https://doi.org/10.3748 wjg.v20.i22.6759.

51 K. Occhipinti and J. W. Smith, 'Irritable bowel syndrome: A reviev and update', *Clinics in Colon and Rectal Surgery*, 25(1), March 2012 pp. 46–52, https://doi.org/10.1055/s-0032-1301759.

52 Ibid.

53 A. S. van Lanen et al., 'Efficacy of a low-FODMAP diet in adu irritable bowel syndrome: a systematic review and meta-analysis *European Journal of Nutrition*, 60(6), September 2021, pp. 3505–2: https://doi.org/10.1007/s00394-020-02473-0. Erratum in: *Europea Journal of Nutrition*, June 2021.

54 A. C. Ford et al., 'ACG Task Force on Management of Irritabl Bowel Syndrome: American College of Gastroenterology Monc graph on Management of Irritable Bowel Syndrome', *America Journal of Gastroenterology*, 113(2), June 2018, pp. 1–18, https://do org/10.1038/s41395-018-0084-x.

55 L. Saha (2014).

56 K. V. Lambeau and J. W. McRorie Jr, 'Fiber supplements and clin cally proven health benefits: How to recognize and recommend a effective fiber therapy', *Journal of the American Association of Nur.*

Practitioners, 29(4), April 2017, pp. 216–23, https://doi.org/10.1002/2327-6924.12447.

57 M. Shoaib et al., 'Inulin: Properties, health benefits and food applications', *Carbohydrate Polymers*, 147, August 2016, pp. 444–54, https://doi.org/10.1016/j.carbpol.2016.04.020.

58 P. Angoorani et al., 'Gut microbiota modulation as a possible mediating mechanism for fasting-induced alleviation of metabolic complications: A systematic review', *Nutrition & Metabolism*, 18(1), December 2021, p. 105, https://doi.org/10.1186/s12986-021-00635-3.

59 G. Li et al., 'Intermittent Fasting Promotes White Adipose Browning and Decreases Obesity by Shaping the Gut Microbiota', *Cell Metabolism*, 26(4), October 2017, pp. 672–85, https://doi.org/10.1016/j.cmet.2017.08.019. Erratum in: *Cell Metabolism*, 26(5), November 2017, p. 801.

60 D. McDonald et al., 'American Gut: An Open Platform for Citizen Science Microbiome Research', *mSystems*, 3(3), May 2018, e00031–18, https://doi.org/10.1128/mSystems.00031-18.

Depression and Dementia: Feeding Your Feelings

1 'The cost of diagnosed mental health conditions: statistics', Mental Health Foundation, https://www.mentalhealth.org.uk/explore-mental-health-statistics/cost-diagnosed-mental-health-conditions-statistics.

2 WHO Depression Fact Sheet, 2017.

3 WHO, *Depression and Other Common Mental Disorders: Global Health Estimates*, Geneva, World Health Organization, 2017, pp. 1–24.

4 I. Lazarevich et al., 'Depression and food consumption in Mexican college students', *Nutricion Hospitalaria*, 35(3), May 2018, pp. 620–6, https://doi.org/10.20960/nh.1500.

5 W. K. Simmons et al., 'Appetite changes reveal depression subgroups with distinct endocrine, metabolic, and immune states', *Molecular Psychiatry*, 25(7), July 2020, pp. 1457–68, https://doi.org/10.1038/s41380-018-0093-6.

6 W. K. Simmons et al., 'Depression-Related Increases and Decreases in Appetite: Dissociable Patterns of Aberrant Activity in Reward and Interoceptive Neurocircuitry', *American Journal of Psychiatry*, 173(4), April 2016, pp. 418–28, https://doi.org/10.1176/appi.ajp.2015.15020162.

7 J. Firth et al., 'The Effects of Dietary Improvement on Symptoms of Depression and Anxiety: A Meta-Analysis of Randomized Controlled Trials', *Psychosomatic Medicine*, 81(3), 2019, pp. 265–80, https://doi.org/10.1097/PSY.0000000000000673

8 M. P. Pase et al., 'Sugary beverage intake and preclinical Alzheimer's disease in the community', *Alzheimer's & Dementia*, 13(9), September 2017, pp. 955–64, https://doi.org/10.1016/j.jalz.2017.01.024.

9 S. Sen et al., 'Serum brain-derived neurotrophic factor, depression, and antidepressant medications: meta-analyses and implications', *Biological Psychiatry*, 64(6), September 2008, pp. 527–32, https://doi.org/10.1016/j.biopsych.2008.05.005.

10 Y. Altuntaş, 'Postprandial Reactive Hypoglycemia', *Sisli Etfal Hastan Tip Bul*, 53(3), August 2019, pp. 215–20, https://doi.org/10.14744/SEMB.2019.59455.

11 A. Menke et al., 'Prevalence of and Trends in Diabetes Among Adults in the United States, 1988–2012', *JAMA*, 314(10), September 2015, pp. 1021–9, https://doi.org/10.1001/jama.2015.10029.

12 S. Penckofer et al., 'Does glycemic variability impact mood and quality of life?', *Diabetes Technology & Therapeutics*, 14(4), April 2012, pp. 303–10, https://doi.org/10.1089/dia.2011.0191.

13 D. Hu et al., 'Sugar-sweetened beverages consumption and the risk of depression: A meta-analysis of observational studies', *Journal of Affective Disorders*, 245, February 2019, pp. 348–55, https://doi.org/10.1016/j.jad.2018.11.015.

14 A. Knüppel et al., 'Sugar intake from sweet food and beverages, common mental disorder and depression: Prospective findings from the Whitehall II study', *Scientific Reports*, 7(1), July 2017, p. 6287, https://doi.org/10.1038/s41598-017-05649-7.

15 G. N. Lindseth et al., 'Neurobehavioral effects of aspartame consumption', *Research in Nursing & Health*, 37(3), June 2014, pp. 185–93, https://doi.org/10.1002/nur.21595.

16 M. Reid et al., 'Long-term dietary compensation for added sugar: Effects of supplementary sucrose drinks over a 4-week period', *British Journal of Nutrition*, 97(1), January 2007, pp. 193–203, https://doi.org/10.1017/S0007114507252705; M. Reid et al., 'Effects of sucrose drinks on macronutrient intake, body weight, and mood state in overweight women over 4 weeks', *Appetite*, 55(1), 2010, pp. 130–6, https://doi.org/10.1016/j.appet.2010.05.001.

17 S. O'Neill et al., 'Depression, Is It Treatable in Adults Utilising Dietary Interventions? A Systematic Review of Randomised Controlled Trials', *Nutrients*, 14(7), March 2022, p. 1398, https://doi.org/10.3390/nu14071398.

18 F. N. Jacka et al., 'A randomised controlled trial of dietary improvement for adults with major depression (the "SMILES" trial)', *BMC Medicine*, 15(1), January 2017, p. 23, https://doi.org/10.1186/s12916-017-0791-y. Erratum in: *BMC Medicine*, 16(1), December 2018, p. 236.

19 G. Lindseth et al., 'The effects of dietary tryptophan on affective disorders', *Archives of Psychiatric Nursing*, 29(2), April 2015, pp. 102–7, https://doi.org/10.1016/j.apnu.2014.11.008.

20 J. E. Alpert and M. Fava, 'Nutrition and depression: The role of folate', *Nutrition Reviews*, 55(5), May 1997, pp. 145–9, https://doi.org/10.1111/j.1753-4887.1997.tb06468.x.

21 M. A. Beydoun et al., 'Serum folate, vitamin B-12, and homocysteine and their association with depressive symptoms among U.S. adults' *Psychosomatic Medicine*, 72(9), November 2010, pp. 862–73, https://doi.org/10.1097/PSY.0b013e3181f61863.

22 M. Park et al., 'Flavonoid-Rich Orange Juice Intake and Altered Gut Microbiome in Young Adults with Depressive Symptom: A Randomized Controlled Study', *Nutrients*, 12(6), June 2020, p. 1815, https://doi.org/10.3390/nu12061815.

23 R. Nair and A. Maseeh, 'Vitamin D: The "sunshine" vitamin', *Journal of Pharmacology & Pharmatherapeutics*, 3(2), April 2012, pp. 118–26, https://doi.org/10.4103/0976-500X.95506.

24 M. F. Holick and T. C. Chen, 'Vitamin D deficiency: a worldwide problem with health consequences', *American Journal of Clinical Nutrition*, 87(4), April 2008, pp. 1080S–6S, https://doi.org/10.1093/ajcn/87.4.1080S.

25 C. Oudshoorn et al., 'Higher serum vitamin D3 levels are associated with better cognitive test performance in patients with Alzheimer's disease', *Dementia and Geriatric Cognitive Disorders*, 25(6), July 2008, pp. 539–43, https://doi.org/10.1159/000134382.

26 D. J. Armstrong et al., 'Vitamin D deficiency is associated with anxiety and depression in fibromyalgia', *Clinical Rheumatology*, 26(4), April 2007, pp. 551–4, https://doi.org/10.1007/s10067-006-0348-5.

27 J. W. Newcomer et al., 'NMDA receptor function, memory, and brain aging', *Dialogues in Clinical Neuroscience*, 2(3), September 2000, pp. 219–32, https://doi.org/10.31887/DCNS.2000.2.3/jnewcomer.

28 G. K. Schwalfenberg and S. J. Genuis, 'The Importance of Magnesium in Clinical Healthcare', *Scientifica* (Cairo), 2017, article 4179326, https://doi.org/10.1155/2017/4179326.

29 G. A. Eby and K. L. Eby, 'Rapid recovery from major depression using magnesium treatment', Medical Hypotheses, 67(2), 2006, pp. 362–70, https://doi.org/10.1016/j.mehy.2006.01.047.

30 D. Phelan et al., 'Magnesium and mood disorders: systematic review and meta-analysis', *BJPsych Open*, 4(4), July 2018, pp. 167–179, https://doi.org/10.1192/bjo.2018.22.

31 U. Tinggi, 'Selenium: its role as antioxidant in human health', *Environmental Health and Preventive Medicine*, 13(2), March 2008, pp. 102–8, https://doi.org/10.1007/s12199-007-0019-4.

32 E. Kesse-Guyot et al., 'French adults' cognitive performance after daily supplementation with antioxidant vitamins and minerals at nutritional doses: a post hoc analysis of the Supplementation in Vitamins and Mineral Antioxidants (SU.VI.MAX) trial', *American*

Journal of Clinical Nutrition, 94(3), September 2011, pp. 892–9, https://doi.org/10.3945/ajcn.110.007815.

33 U. Tinggi (2008).

34 S. S. Sajjadi, et al., 'The role of selenium in depression: a systematic review and meta-analysis of human observational and interventional studies', *Scientific Reports* 12, article 1045 (2022), https://doi.org/10.1038/s41598-022-05078-1

35 P. D. Chilibeck et al., 'Effect of creatine supplementation during resistance training on lean tissue mass and muscular strength in older adults: a meta-analysis', *Open Access Journal of Sports Medicine*, 8 November 2017, pp. 213–26, https://doi.org/10.2147/OAJSM.S123529.

36 I. K. Lyoo et al., 'A randomized, double-blind placebo-controlled trial of oral creatine monohydrate augmentation for enhanced response to a selective serotonin reuptake inhibitor in women with major depressive disorder', *American Journal of Psychiatry*, 169(9), September 2012, pp. 937–45, https://doi.org/10.1176/appi.ajp.2012.12010009.

37 I. K. Lyoo et al., 'Multinuclear magnetic resonance spectroscopy of high-energy phosphate metabolites in human brain following oral supplementation of creatine-monohydrate', *Psychiatry Research: Neuroimaging*, 123(2), June 2003, pp. 87–100, https://doi.org/10.1016/s0925-4927(03)00046-5.

38 M. J. Siddiqui et al., '(*Crocus sativus* L.) as an Antidepressant', *Journal of Pharmacy & BioAllied Sciences*, 10(4), October–December 2018, pp. 173–180, https://doi.org/10.4103/JPBS.JPBS_83_18.

39 W. Marx et al., 'Effect of saffron supplementation on symptoms of depression and anxiety: a systematic review and meta-analysis', *Nutrition Reviews*, 77(8), August 2019, pp. 557–71, https://doi.org/10.1093/nutrit/nuz023.

40 H. S. Lee et al., 'Psychiatric disorders risk in patients with iron deficiency anemia and association with iron supplementation medications: A nationwide database analysis', *BMC Psychiatry*, 20(1), May 2020, p. 216, https://doi.org/10.1186/s12888-020-02621-0.

41 L. Fusar-Poli et al., 'Curcumin for depression: A meta-analysis', *Critical Reviews in Food Science and Nutrition*, 60(15), 2020, pp. 2643–53, https://doi.org/10.1080/10408398.2019.1653260.

42 G. Grosso et al., 'Coffee, tea, caffeine and risk of depression: A systematic review and dose-response meta-analysis of observational studies', *Molecular Nutrition & Food Research*, 60(1), January 2016, pp. 223–4, https://doi.org/10.1002/mnfr.201500620.

43 L. Klevebrant and A. Frick, 'Effects of caffeine on anxiety and panic attacks in patients with panic disorder: A systematic review and meta-analysis', *General Hospital Psychiatry*, 74, 2022, pp. 22–31, https://doi.org/10.1016/j.genhosppsych.2021.11.005.

44 M. A. Petrilli et al., 'The Emerging Role for Zinc in Depression and Psychosis', *Frontiers in Pharmacology*, 8, June 2017, p. 414, https://doi.org/10.3389/fphar.2017.00414.

45 S. Yosaee et al., 'Zinc in depression: From development to treatment: A comparative/ dose response meta-analysis of observational studies and randomized controlled trials', *General Hospital Psychiatry*, 74, 2022, pp. 110–117, https://doi.org/10.1016/j.genhosppsych.2020.08.001.

46 Y. Xu, 'Role of dietary factors in the prevention and treatment for depression: An umbrella review of meta-analyses of prospective studies', *Translational Psychiatry*, 11(1), September 2021, https://pubmed.ncbi.nlm.nih.gov/34531367/.

47 J. L. Cummings et al., 'Alzheimer's disease drug-development pipeline: few candidates, frequent failures', *Alzheimer's Research & Therapy*, 6(4), July 2014, p. 37, https://doi.org/10.1186/alzrt269.

48 H. Li et al., 'Association of Ultraprocessed Food Consumption with Risk of Dementia: A Prospective Cohort', *Neurology*, July 2022, https://doi.org/10.1212/WNL.0000000000200871.

49 S. M. de la Monte and M. Tong, 'Mechanisms of nitrosamine-mediated neurodegeneration: potential relevance to sporadic Alzheimer's disease', *Journal of Alzheimer's Disease*, 17(4), 2009, pp. 817–25, https://doi.org/10.3233/JAD-2009-1098.

50 For example, this study on 830 healthy adults showed that high blood glucose was related to poorer overall performance on perceptual speed, greater rates of decline in cognitive function and higher glycaemic loads related to overall worse cognitive performance. S. Seetharaman et al., 'Blood glucose, diet-based glycemic load and cognitive aging among dementia-free older adults', *The Journals of Gerontology. Series A, Biological Sciences and Medical Sciences*, 70(4), April 2015, pp. 471–9, https://doi.org/10.1093/gerona/glu135; S. I. Sünram-Lea and L. Owen, 'The impact of diet-based glycaemic response and glucose regulation on cognition: Evidence across the lifespan', *Proceedings of the Nutrition Society*, 76(4), November 2017, pp. 466–77, https://doi.org/10.1017/S0029665117000829; M. Gentreau et al., 'High Glycemic Load Is Associated with Cognitive Decline in Apolipoprotein E ε4 Allele Carriers', *Nutrients*, 12(12), November 2020, p. 3619, https://doi.org/10.3390/nu12123619.

51 M. K. Taylor et al., 'A high-glycemic diet is associated with cerebral amyloid burden in cognitively normal older adults', *American Journal of Clinical Nutrition*, 106(6), December 2017, pp. 1463–70, https://doi.org/10.3945/ajcn.117.162263; K. M. Rodrigue et al., 'β-Amyloid burden in healthy aging: regional distribution and cognitive consequences', *Neurology*, 78(6), February 2012, pp. 387–95, https://doi.org/10.1212/WNL.0b013e318245d295.

52 I. V. Kurochkin et al., 'Insulin-Degrading Enzyme in the Fight against Alzheimer's Disease', *Trends in Pharmacolological Sciences*, 39(1), January 2018, pp. 49–58, https://doi.org/10.1016/j.tips.2017.10.008.

53 B. S. Lennerz et al., 'Effects of dietary glycemic index on brain regions related to reward and craving in men', *American Journal of Clinical Nutrition*, 98(3), September 2013, pp. 641–7, https://doi.org/10.3945/ajcn.113.064113.

54 E. A. Maguire et al., 'Navigation-related structural change in the hippocampi of taxi drivers', *Proceedings of the National Academy of Sciences of the United States of America*, 97(8), April 2000, pp. 4398–403, https://doi.org/10.1073/pnas.070039597.

55 R. Molteni et al., 'A high-fat, refined sugar diet reduces hippocampal brain-derived neurotrophic factor, neuronal plasticity, and learning', *Neuroscience*, 112(4), 2002, pp. 803–14, https://doi.org/10.1016/s0306-4522(02)00123-9.

56 C. Willmann et al., 'Insulin sensitivity predicts cognitive decline in individuals with prediabetes', *BMJ Open Diabetes Research & Care*, 8(2), November 2020, e001741, https://doi.org/10.1136/bmjdrc-2020-001741.

57 I. Hajjar et al., 'Oxidative stress predicts cognitive decline with aging in healthy adults: An observational study', *Journal of Neuroinflammation*, 15(1), January 2018, p. 17, https://doi.org/10.1186/s12974-017-1026-z.

58 I. E. Orhan et al., 'Flavonoids and dementia: An update', *Current Medicinal Chemistry*, 22(8), 2015, pp. 1004–15, https://doi.org/10.2174/0929867322666141212122352.

59 J. P. Spencer et al., 'Neuroinflammation: modulation by flavonoids and mechanisms of action', *Molecular Aspects of Medicine*, 33(1), February 2012, pp. 83–97, https://doi.org/10.1016/j.mam.2011.10.016.

60 R. J. Williams and J. P. Spencer, 'Flavonoids, cognition, and dementia: Actions, mechanisms, and potential therapeutic utility for Alzheimer disease', *Free Radical Biology and Medicine*, 52(1), January 2012, pp. 35–45, https://doi.org/10.1016/j.freeradbiomed.2011.09.010.

61 L. Letenneur et al., 'Flavonoid intake and cognitive decline over a 10-year period', *American Journal of Epidemiology*, 165(12), June 2007, pp. 1364–71, https://doi.org/10.1093/aje/kwm036.

62 E. E. Devore et al., 'Dietary intakes of berries and flavonoids in relation to cognitive decline', *Annals of Neurology*, 72(1), July 2012, pp. 135–43, https://doi.org/10.1002/ana.23594.

63 C. Cui et al., 'Effects of soy isoflavones on cognitive function: A systematic review and meta-analysis of randomized controlled trials', *Nutrition Reviews*, 78(2), February 2020, pp. 134–44, https://doi.org/10.1093/nutrit/nuz050.

64 R. Krikorian et al., 'Blueberry supplementation improves memory in older adults', *Journal of Agricultural and Food Chemistry*, 58(7), April 2010, pp. 3996–4000, https://doi.org/10.1021/jf9029332.

65 D. J. Lamport et al., 'Concord grape juice, cognitive function, and driving performance: a 12-wk, placebo-controlled, randomized crossover trial in mothers of preteen children', *American Journal of Clinical Nutrition*, 103(3), March 2016, pp. 775–83, https://doi.org/10.3945/ajcn.115.114553.

66 A. R. Whyte and C. M. Williams, 'Effects of a single dose of a flavonoid-rich blueberry drink on memory in 8 to 10 y old children', *Nutrition*, 31(3), March 2015, pp. 531–4, https://doi.org/10.1016/j.nut.2014.09.013.

67 A. S. Abdelhamid et al., 'Omega-3 fatty acids for the primary and secondary prevention of cardiovascular disease', *Cochrane Database of Systematic Reviews*, 3(3), February 2020, CD003177, https://doi.org/10.1002/14651858.CD003177.pub5.

68 C. Sahlin et al., 'Docosahexaenoic acid stimulates non-amyloidogenic APP processing resulting in reduced Abeta levels in cellular models of Alzheimer's disease', *European Journal of Neuroscience*, 26(4), August 2007, pp. 882–9, https://doi.org/10.1111/j.1460-9568.2007.05719.x.

69 M. Oksman et al., 'Impact of different saturated fatty acid, polyunsaturated fatty acid and cholesterol containing diets on beta-amyloid accumulation in APP/PS1 transgenic mice', *Neurobiology of Disease*, 23(3), September 2006, pp. 563–72, https://doi.org/10.1016/j.nbd.2006.04.013.

70 C. N. Serhan et al., 'Resolvins, docosatrienes, and neuroprotectins, novel omega-3-derived mediators, and their endogenous aspirin-triggered epimers', *Lipids*, November 2004, 39(11), pp. 1125–32, https://doi.org/10.1007/s11745-004-1339-7.

71 Y. Papanikolaou et al., 'U.S. adults are not meeting recommended levels for fish and omega-3 fatty acid intake: results of an analysis using observational data from NHANES 2003–2008', *Nutrition Journal*, 13, April 2014, p. 31, https://doi.org/10.1186/1475-2891-13-31. Erratum in: ibid., p. 64.

72 H. Gerster, 'Can adults adequately convert alpha-linolenic acid (18:3n-3) to eicosapentaenoic acid (20:5n-3) and docosahexaenoic

acid (22:6n-3)', *International Journal for Vitamin and Nutrition Research*, 68(3), 1998, pp. 159–73, https://pubmed.ncbi.nlm.nih.gov/9637947.

73 Y. Zhang et al., 'Intakes of fish and polyunsaturated fatty acids and mild-to-severe cognitive impairment risks: a dose-response meta-analysis of 21 cohort studies', *American Journal of Clinical Nutrition*, 103(2), February 2016, pp. 330–40, https://doi.org/10.3945/ajcn.115.124081.

74 M. C. Morris et al., 'Association of Seafood Consumption, Brain Mercury Level, and APOE ε4 Status with Brain Neuropathology in Older Adults', *JAMA*, February 2016, 315(5), pp. 489–97, https://doi.org/10.1001/jama.2015.19451.

75 G. Mazereeuw et al., 'Effects of ω-3 fatty acids on cognitive performance: A meta-analysis', *Neurobiology of Aging*, 33(7), July 2012, p. 1482.e17–29, https://doi.org/10.1016/j.neurobiolaging.2011.12.014.

76 F. Araya-Quintanilla et al., 'Effectiveness of omega-3 fatty acid supplementation in patients with Alzheimer disease: A systematic review and meta-analysis', *Neurologia* (English edn), 35(2), March 2020, pp. 105–14, https://doi.org/10.1016/j.nrl.2017.07.009.

77 M. Moss and L. Oliver, 'Plasma 1,8-cineole correlates with cognitive performance following exposure to rosemary essential oil aroma', *Therapeutic Advances in Psychopharmacology*, 2(3), June 2012, pp. 103–13, https://doi.org/10.1177/2045125312436573.

78 M. T. Islam et al., 'Immunomodulatory Effects of Diterpenes and Their Derivatives Through NLRP3 Inflammasome Pathway: A Review', *Frontiers in Immunology*, 11, September 2020, 572136, https://doi.org/10.3389/fimmu.2020.572136. Erratum in: *Frontiers in Immunology*, 12, April 2021, 692302.

79 W. Sayorwan et al., 'Effects of inhaled rosemary oil on subjective feelings and activities of the nervous system', *Scientia Pharmaceutica*, 81(2), 2013, pp. 531–42, https://doi.org/10.3797/scipharm.1209-05.

80 Q. P. Liu et al., 'Habitual coffee consumption and risk of cognitive decline/dementia: A systematic review and meta-analysis of prospective cohort studies', *Nutrition*, 32(6), June 2016, pp. 628–36; S. L. Gardener et al., 'Higher Coffee Consumption Is Associated With

Slower Cognitive Decline and Less Cerebral Aβ-Amyloid Accumulation Over 126 Months: Data From the Australian Imaging, Biomarkers, and Lifestyle Study', *Frontiers in Aging Neuroscience*, 13, November 2021, 744872, https://doi.org/10.3389/fnagi.2021.744872.

81 J. Lorenzo Calvo et al., 'Caffeine and Cognitive Functions in Sports: A Systematic Review and Meta-Analysis', *Nutrients*, 13(3), March 2021, p. 868, https://doi.org/10.3390/nu13030868.

82 C. Doepker et al., 'Key Findings and Implications of a Recent Systematic Review of the Potential Adverse Effects of Caffeine Consumption in Healthy Adults, Pregnant Women, Adolescents, and Children', *Nutrients*, 10(10), October 2018, p. 1536, https://doi.org/10.3390/nu10101536.

83 R. Poole et al., 'Coffee consumption and health: Umbrella review of meta-analyses of multiple health outcomes', *BMJ*, 359, November 2017, https://doi.org/10.1136/bmj.j5024. Erratum in: *BMJ*, 360, January 2018, k194.

84 G. Schepici et al., 'Ginger, a Possible Candidate for the Treatment of Dementias?', *Molecules*, 26(18), September 2021, p. 5700, https://doi.org/10.3390/molecules26185700.

85 N. Saenghong et al., '*Zingiber officinale* Improves Cognitive Function of the Middle-Aged Healthy Women', *Evidence-Based Complementary and Alternative Medicine*, 2012, 383062, https://doi.org/10.1155/2012/383062.

86 R. Lakhan et al., 'The Role of Vitamin E in Slowing Down Mild Cognitive Impairment: A Narrative Review', *Healthcare* (Basel), 9(11), November 2021, p. 1573, https://doi.org/10.3390/healthcare9111573.

87 J. H. Kang et al., 'A randomized trial of vitamin E supplementation and cognitive function in women', *Archives of Internal Medicine*, 166(22), December 2006, pp. 2462–8, https://doi.org/10.1001/archinte.166.22.2462.

88 E. Leclerc et al., 'The effect of caloric restriction on working memory in healthy non-obese adults', *CNS Spectrums*, 25(1), February 2020, pp. 2–8, https://doi.org/10.1017/S1092852918001566.

89 W. Lü et al., 'Effects of dietary restriction on cognitive function: A systematic review and meta-analysis', *Nutritional Neuroscience*, April 2022, pp. 1–11, https://doi.org/10.1080/1028415X.2022.2068876.

90 R. Daviet, 'Associations between alcohol consumption and gray and white matter volumes in the UK Biobank', *Nature Communications*, 13(1), 2022, p. 1175, https://doi.org/10.1038/s41467-022-28735-5.

91 M. C. Morris et al., 'MIND diet slows cognitive decline with aging', *Alzheimer's & Dementia*, 11(9), September 2015, pp. 1015–22, https://doi.org/10.1016/j.jalz.2015.04.011. Epub 15 June 2015.

92 D. E. Hosking et al., 'MIND not Mediterranean diet related to 12-year incidence of cognitive impairment in an Australian longitudinal cohort study', *Alzheimer's & Dementia*, 15(4), April 2019, pp. 581–9, https://doi.org/10.1016/j.jalz.2018.12.011.

93 S. Kheirouri and M. Alizadeh, 'MIND diet and cognitive performance in older adults: A systematic review', *Critical Reviews in Food Science and Nutrition*, 14, May 2021, pp. 1–19, https://doi.org/10.1080/10408398.2021.1925220.

Appendix: Hierarchy of Evidence

1 D. B. Resnik and K. C. Elliott, 'Taking financial relationships into account when assessing research', *Accountability in Research*, 20(3), 2013, pp. 184–205, https://doi.org/10.1080/08989621.2013.788383.

2 L. K. John et al., 'Effect of revealing authors' conflicts of interests in peer review: randomized controlled trial', *BMJ*, 367, November 2019, l5896, https://doi.org/10.1136/bmj.l5896.

Index

Index